NUTRITION DESTINATION

NUTRITION DESTINATION

Put The Power Of Food Into Your Hands
Through Your Fitness Journey

DANI KEPERLING

Nutrition Destination: Put the Power of Food Into Your Own Hands Through Your Fitness Journey

ISBN: 978-0-578-28308-190000

For more information or would like to contact me. Visit www.bedanifit.com

Acknowledgment

This book wouldn't be possible without the support of Matt, Noah, Marley, Hadley, and many supportive family and friends.

Table of Contents

Introduction 13

Method # 1: Bridging the Gap Between Nutrition & Fitness......17

Method # 2: The Right Mindset 21

Method # 3: Your Best Nutrition Plan Starts with Your BMR ...33

Method # 4: Eating for Your Specific Fitness Goal 39

Fitness Goal: Strength or Weight Training 43

Fitness Goal: Total Body Conditioning 55

Fitness Goal: Cardiovascular Fitness 65

Fitness Goal: Functional Movement & Flexibility.....................81

Meal Break-Down, Timing & Tracking...87

Method # 5: Water, Hydration Needs, & Water Jug Challenge ..97

Method # 6: Bring Your Fitness and Nutrition Goals Home.......105

Plateaus Are Actually Good 109

Living Your Best Life...112

Appendix A: Dani's Food Go-To's 114

Appendix B: My Food Go-To's 122

BONUS
Support & Accountability!

Thank you for purchasing my book Nutrition Destination—Put the Power of Food into your Hands Through your Fitness Journey.

We are not meant to reach our destination alone!

I've created a community specific to this book to provide support and accountability on Facebook. Visit my website and subscribe to receive weekly emails for tips, strategies, recipes, exercise demos and more!

Scan the QR Code to follow me and join the community.

Join the Community   Be Dani Fit Website   Dani's Instagram

If you've found this book helpful, please post a review on Amazon so others may find it.

Advance Praise

"Dani has been a much-needed and welcomed inspiration, challenging me to challenge myself. Her compassion, drive, and dedication to spread health and wellness are genuine. She has been a crucial part in educating me to understand the effects of carbs, fats, and proteins, as well as guiding me to find my pursuit of healthiness. For that, I am forever grateful!"

~ Lisa Hager

"Dani has taught me how to eat, what to eat, and when to eat to take my health and fitness to the next level. It's about learning to listen to your body, feeding what it needs to do what you want it to do. If you are not eating right, you won't get results. And it's not about strict dieting. It is about planning and properly fueling your body."

~ Ray Zdradzinski

"Having a coach like Dani to teach me proper nutrition and fitness principles to live by day-to-day has helped me influence others around me, who are not health and fitness conscious, to live a better life."

~ Steve Gehris

"Dani makes losing weight feel easy. As long as you stick to the plan the results are guaranteed."

~ Vance Yacomes

"I cannot speak highly enough of Dani Keperling! Dani's fitness and nutrition knowledge has undoubtedly been developed from her years of education, training, and experience. She not only helped me prepare for my first bodybuilding competition but also continued to be my coach for over a year due to multiple show cancellations. Throughout the entire process, she continued to help me adjust my diet and exercise routines and helped me keep a positive mindset through difficult times. Her knowledge and friendship are invaluable!"

~Brooke Hatfield

"The biggest and hardest lesson I learned from Dani on my fitness journey is that food is fuel, and carbs are not scary! As someone who struggled with weight and eating disorders, it was hard to break the calorie counting and eat a sweet potato! Once I trusted her process, I was able to make progress and maintain a healthy, happy lifestyle in the gym and kitchen."

~ Kelly Gerrity-Haldeman

"Working with Dani on my nutrition has helped me to understand the importance of healthy foods and how to adjust the amount of food to eat properly for my fitness goals. I was skeptical about the process—tracking calories, measuring out food, and how to get fit in general. I'm grateful she went the extra mile to help and stick with me on the road to a fit lifestyle. I lost over fifty pounds and decided to compete in a bodybuilding competition which she coached me through!"

~ Mario Banda-Pito

"I've always been an athlete. I played team sports all of my life but neglected to realize how my nutrition played a major role in my overall fitness and health. Dani taught me about meal timing, how to eat to fuel my workouts, and how to be consistent with both nutrition and my workouts. Before I adopted Dani's methods, I thought I was eating healthy, but in reality, I was not. I'm so glad I took the time to learn about nutrition and how to eat. Not only have I lost weight, but I also built muscle and decreased body fat. I am healthier and stronger thanks to Dani's knowledge of nutrition!"

~ Rachael Hasselhan

"Dani builds a nutrition plan that fits your goals. Her plan not only helps you achieve your fitness goals, but helps you live a healthier life overall."

~ Johanna Arias

INTRODUCTION
Fit versus Healthy

Use this book as your primary training tool to equip your fit lifestyle. Notice that I used the word *fit,* not healthy. The reason is that the meaning of the word healthy is so subjective and vague now. I bet, if you were to ask your friends and family, most would consider themselves as healthy or somewhat healthy—does that mean what they eat, how active they are, their hygiene, their mental state, or what? But if you ask them if they would consider themselves fit, how many would say yes?

It's sad to say, but society has downplayed the meaning of the word healthy to justify eating crap that seems like the healthier version of a product that would be declared unhealthy. There are so many varieties of snack chips out there. If you're opting for a *low-fat* version and consider yourself healthy, I'm sorry; you've been scammed, just like most people. Trust me, don't trust the advertising from companies. Take a look at the ingredients, not just what the packaging claims to be true. Believe it or not, sometimes the healthy snack ingredients are worse than the original because they need to add filler back into the product from whatever they took out to make it still appealing and taste good. My point is that switching from one processed product to another does not make you healthier. You should focus on scaling back from many processed products altogether and implement changes that incorporate less processed foods. The ingredients are essential when it comes to your health!

You will find that more and more companies portray certain foods as healthy and are remarkably creative when marketing junk food as healthy in grocery and convenience stores. Unfortunately, when we make one of these *sensible* choices, we pat ourselves on the back. By no means am I going to belittle anyone who falls for these gimmicks. As consumers, we need to do a better job at digging deeper than reading the catchy label on the front—we need to look at the ingredients behind the label.

However, being uninformed and making a decision based on persuasion and current knowledge is definitely different from knowing better but making poor choices. Let's call a spade a spade. Processed food, claimed to be healthy or not, is still processed. There's room in your diet for it, but it shouldn't make up the majority of the foods you eat on a daily basis.

Let's take a look at the word *fit*. According to the dictionary; as an adjective, fit means having the requisite qualities or skills to undertake something competently; as a verb, fit means to be of the right shape and size for something; as a noun, fit is the particular way in which a thing matches something else. The meaning of fit is so much more than what usually comes to mind—an athletic person with a muscular build. That's great if that's your ultimate goal. However, having a muscular body isn't the only thing that makes a person well-rounded in their fitness.

Fit versus Healthy

Your fitness should cover the following: your mindset, activity and fitness goals, your nutrition, getting enough rest to recharge your body, and your perseverance and determination through life's challenges. If you've ever struggled with any of those aspects I have just listed or have felt that you've been held back in becoming the best version of yourself, then this book is for you.

METHOD # 1:
Bridging the Gap Between Nutrition & Fitness

Empowerment is the process of becoming stronger and more confident, especially in controlling one's life and claiming one's rights. It is your right to know the power of food and how to use food to fuel your lifestyle, no matter how many times or ways it may change through your lifetime. Understanding the why behind the diet will give you the power to choose whether it's right for you or not. There are different eating styles that work, so why do people experience so many failures?

We are not failures. The diet has failed us. I'm not saying diets can't work, but most diets out there don't talk about or focus on a person's mindset or use their fitness goals as the driving force behind the diet itself. There are cracks in fad diets, and it's only a matter of time until we fall through. Diet plans that give food restrictions or cut out food groups altogether eventually lose momentum, especially if you want to start eating the restrictive foods again or if you have been eating below your daily caloric needs.

The number of calories you should consume differs from person to person. There are factors to consider to figure out how much you should be eating daily, like age, gender, height, weight, and body fat, which

I will talk about in the next chapter. Any diet that doesn't consider any of the components I discussed will fail—it's a matter of when. Then what? Back to square one in the hope of finding something that works.

I like to challenge people with a question when they are thinking about going on a particular diet—Does your plan have your fitness goal in mind? That is not the same as the diet suggesting that you add exercise to make the diet more effective. Your nutrition should not be treated as a separate entity from your activity and fitness goals. Ultimately, our activity should drive our nutrition and what we eat. Frequently, physical activity is skipped over entirely or considered secondary compared to nutrition. So here's the thing—fueling your body with what it actually needs based on the activity and exercise you do will produce the greatest results.

How do I know that? Because I have been living out that testimony since 2006. Not only do I have the education to back up what I believe about fitness and nutrition, but I have put all of my methods to the test by helping myself and my clients over the years. I can confidently say I can make my body look any way I want it to using different means of exercise and nutrition. I am not saying that arrogantly, so please don't get the wrong idea. My practical methods are just that effective and successful.

You're probably thinking, "Well, this girl doesn't drink or have fun"—I do. "She probably doesn't have kids to ruin and stress out her body"—I have three, two girls and a step-son. "She has hours to spend at the gym"—I don't, and I homeschool two out of three of our kids. My methods are truly practical, and if you're intentional, you will get there too.

Let's look at athletes—from marathoners, team sports, and bodybuilders—all are intentional with their diet and exercise. Their nutrition plan is based on the physical activity they perform. The evidence is out there that proper nutrition improves function, performance, immunity, and well-being of the body. Performance may not be important to you, but function, immunity, and well-being should be! For athletes, it's not unheard of to have an off-season and an in-season diet. Why? Because their training and activity change during the year, and what they're eating should too. It makes sense to me!

Think like an athlete! Your athletic ability does not matter. I don't care if you have never played a sport in your life. You don't actually need physical skills—just a mindset like an athlete. Our bodies were meant to move, and if I can motivate you to get in a little activity every day because your nutrition and health depend on it, then so be it.

Something else to keep in mind is to think about nutrition and exercise working as one. Think about New Year's resolutions. From January through March, the gyms are flooded with new people who hope to lose weight. They start exercising and try to get into a routine. Between one and three months, most wonder why they haven't lost any weight. They lose motivation and consistency and make the association that exercise has no positive effect on weight loss.

The fact is that exercise alone, without any dietary changes, can have little effect on body composition; however, there could be an improvement in stamina and strength. Unfortunately, by not changing your nutrition plan that mirrors the exercise you performed and not being intentional with your diet, you may now associate exercise and yourself as failures.

Did you know that many people actually eat more without realizing it when starting a new exercise plan? So even if you're tracking the calories you burn at the gym, you might accidentally take in additional calories that cancel out the calories burned! Some studies have also shown an increase in body weight within the first several months of starting exercise. No wonder exercise can get a bad rap! Who wants to put work into something that feels like it sets you back?

Wrapping your head around the idea that fitness and nutrition affect one another by giving your body what it needs based on what you're doing throughout the day (or what you will be doing) helps you stay intentional with eating and exercising. Making that connection will aid in becoming in-tune with your body in the long run, giving it what it needs and optimizing the results you can see and feel.

You're ready! I can feel it! Where do we start? First, we need to set the tone for the right learning environment. You actually hold that key yourself—it's your mindset.

METHOD # 2:
The Right Mindset

Maybe you're reading this with an optimistic, open mind or perhaps wrestling with feelings of fear, failure, or defeat. I have helped people with different mindsets when starting their fitness and nutrition journey and have seen countless breakthroughs no matter their previous mindset. You may think spending a chapter on mindset sounds silly, but think of it as your *hype* chapter. When you go to a concert, and you've paid hundreds of dollars to see your favorite musical artist or band play, they are not the first ones you hear. There could be a DJ or smaller name bands that will play first to hype up the crowd.

As you read on, I want you to feel more confident about ultimately choosing the way you can eat for the rest of your life and be happy doing it. So, where's your current mindset? Let's keep it simple—do you feel you have a more positive or negative outlook on things and situations?

Remember those personality tests we took when we were younger that tell you if you are a more optimistic—glass-half-full kind of person or a more pessimistic—glass-half-empty kind of person? You could argue that people who have a positive outlook already have an advantage in making positive changes in their lives because they have the right mindset. Of course, I'm not a psychologist—but there could be some truth behind that assumption.

I have made correlations with past clients. People with a positive outlook usually had a growth mindset, and people with a negative outlook had more of a fixed mindset. The most significant difference I've seen between growth mindsets and fixed mindsets is the reaction from which situations and circumstances are interpreted. Once interpreted, the outcome can be very different based on the person's reaction.

I have worked with both the Negative-Nancys and Positive-Pennys in the world with fantastic outcomes. I have discovered that a common factor between the two personalities is the passion behind the cause. People with the will to change, and the passion behind it, will achieve success.

Someone who tends to be more pessimistic or hard on themselves needs the motivation to keep going with smaller wins along the way. In addition, they need to surround themselves with good influences and role models. They can be easily influenced through social media and people in their immediate circle—positive affirmation is essential at every step of their journey.

Those with a more positive outlook look for ways to challenge or grow mentally. They don't let failures define them as a person but take it as an opportunity to learn from the experience. Setting goals and milestones keep them motivated and focused, and they are typically self-driven if given the right tools and support.

No matter your outlook or what type of mindset you think you may have, I know the information in this book can help you, the same way it's helped many of my clients. Our brains are ever-changing, so who says our mindset can't do the same if we have the correct influences driving our success.

The *first* thing you need to do is write out your obstacles—anything that could potentially prevent you from hitting your fitness goals. But did you notice that the first thing wasn't to write out your goal? I'm intentionally speaking to the Negative-Nancys of the world because, most likely, that's where your mind went first—towards the things that would prevent you from achieving your goals.

List out all obstacles that could potentially prevent you from reaching your fitness and nutrition goals, and then write out ways to overcome each obstacle next to it. Then, do the same with your goals.

Next, share these obstacles with a close family member or friend—they are your accountability partner. This person may be one of the solutions to overcome one or all of your obstacles and help you reach your goals.

Obstacle 1:

_____

_____

_____

Obstacle 2:

_____

_____

_____

Obstacle 3:

_____

_____

_____

Short term goal(s)—4-6 weeks:

_____

_____

_____

Short/Long term goal(s)—6-12 weeks:

_____

_____

_____

Long term goal(s)—12-24 weeks:

_____

_____

_____

My accountability partner's name:_____

Date I shared my obstacles with my accountability partner:

__-__-____

The Nancys may say, "I'm ready to change, but—I've always failed at everything. My job is too consuming. I can't cook, so I'll never be able to eat healthily." On the other hand, the Pennys of the world may say something like, "I'm ready to change. I'm ready to try again. This will be good for me. I can do this." Both groups of people are about to learn something new and unfamiliar; however, you can see a very different mindset in each group about starting the program before they have even begun.

You picked up this book because you're done with the dieting games, and you're hopeful about implementing fitness and proper nutritional habits the right way. But, even though you have a different outlook, you share a common factor—the desire to change. So, instead of tackling something new and unfamiliar in the way you usually do and arguing that one person may have an advantage to a successful outcome over another, we will approach it altogether differently.

Think of this as starting a new class in college. I know; I already have red flags going up from some of you. It doesn't matter if you went to college or not or dropped out. None of that matters, and this will not be college-level material or anything intimidating. The reason why I compared it to a college course is that everyone diving into this book has previous knowledge about eating and exercise. I correlate it the same as graduating from high school—some may be more advanced than others, but everyone has basic education on nutrition and fitness. Even if you know the very minimum, you all have been eating food for some time and are aware that food gives you the energy to perform an activity.

No matter what diets you've followed in the past or what crazy things you've eaten to gain weight, lose weight, maintain weight, and everything in between—it still comes down to putting the right amount of fats, proteins, and carbohydrates into your body to get you through your day and achieve a specific outcome. So no matter if you're Positive-Penny or Negative-Nancy, you're all diving into this with the same understanding of what food can do for us. It's my job to teach you how and when to choose the right foods for you, depending on your fitness goal.

Besides not feeling physically fit, have you ever thought you were unfit for a particular role or job? How did that turn out? In that position, you have two options: crumble and fold or pursue and conquer.

I think it's safe to say that we've all been in that position. Even as a kid starting in kindergarten. There are a lot of firsts—the bus, meeting a bunch of new kids, buying lunch, being away from mom and dad all day, relying on ourselves to go to the bathroom on time without having to run while pulling down our pants at the same time! Thank goodness we have to conquer all of those *firsts* when we are young and resilient because, as adults, I don't think we would make it to lunch!

I also know many parents, who have felt unfit to be parents, are some of the best parents I know! When I was a young parent in my late twenties, my husband and I reconnected with our faith and started attending a church. Being disconnected for so long my husband and I were eager to listen and take in the sermons every week.

One evening we attended a church get-together to meet and mingle with other people around the church. We got to know our pastor more through conversation and shared our interest in joining a men's and women's Bible study group because we felt so new to our faith again.

Weeks had passed, then I received an email from the pastor asking if I would help lead the women's ministry for the entire church! He felt I had a lot to offer and wanted my input in creating the women's Bible study for fall and spring sessions. I can honestly say I never felt more unfit for a position.

Up until that point, I had barely read the Bible. I didn't even think I owned one, and now I'm supposed to be in a leading role at church for women's ministry? I had never done a Bible study before. The no-brainer answer would have been, "Thank you, and I'm honored, but I'd like to participate in the study, not lead it."

But I accepted the offer and, feeling like a kindergartner all over again, went into the meeting with a team of strong ladies to start the planning process for our church's women's ministry. (P.S. I made sure I used the bathroom before I went—one less thing to worry about!)

I never felt so ill-equipped and unfit for a role. I knew, going into it, that I probably was the furthest from God out of everyone there. It didn't matter how physically fit I was; mentally, I was the most out-of-shape person there. I needed to start somewhere. I was able to speak and listen to women much wiser than I and realized I needed to take advantage of this chance. At the time, I didn't see the value I had to bring to the group, but this experience was not about how I valued myself; it was an opportunity given to me that I never knew I needed. Eventually, I spoke to over sixty women in a room about my story and unleashed my influence on those around me.

Now, it's your time to unleash that passion for bettering yourself for good! We all have that desire—maybe it's not far from the surface, or perhaps, it may take weeks of digging until you find that spark to ignite it. So, do me a favor while you continue on this journey with me and *Act As If*. . . If I didn't *Act As If*. . . in all of the situations where I felt unfit for a job or role, I wouldn't be where I am today.

I know you're thinking, "You want me to act as if what?" The phrase *Act As If*. . . has gotten me through the most challenging times of my life. I'm not strictly talking about food here—relationships, jobs, everyday life, and the curve balls that have been thrown my way. In other words, even though you have no idea what you're doing, act or pretend as if you do. I'm sure you have heard the phrase *fake it 'til you make it. Act As If*. . . is the same idea. Sometimes you need to convince yourself you are capable. Sometimes you need to own the stage, even though you don't feel worthy of the spotlight. It doesn't matter how confident you might be, there will be times when you think you don't have what it takes, but you're going to need to act like you do and fight like hell for it.

This phrase—*Act As If*. . . is so important to me that I literally have it tattooed on my body. Of course, you don't have to do that, but I know if I did not believe and follow that phrase, my life would have taken a very different path, and that is an entirely different book I'll have to write. Whenever I'm faced with an *Act As If*. . . situation, I typically go through specific steps from the start of the first encounter, leading me through to the end. I've laid out the steps to take below:

Step 1: You will *act as if* you are capable of changing your nutritional and fitness habits. Failure is not an option. Set your doubts aside, and make a believer out of yourself.

Step 2: You will start *doing* things to change your nutritional and fitness habits, even if it pushes you out of your comfort zone. If you don't do something that will get you closer to your goal because you don't think you can or if you fear failure, you're back to the first step of acting as if you are capable. Without this first step, you won't successfully be able to move forward.

Step 3: You will start *believing* in the changes—truly believing! We are done acting by now, and the *doing* step will get easier. By now, you are leaving old habits in the dust and creating new habits. This step reinforces the second step, telling you that what you're doing will make a difference.

Step 4: Finally, you will be *accomplishing* things you never thought you were capable of doing. The fourth step is also a time to reflect on the challenges you had on the journey to your goal and see how far you've come. Depending on how big the challenges you've overcome or goals met, the fourth step can be the confidence-booster you need to keep going.

I wish I could tell you a timeline for each step, but that will be entirely up to you and what the universe throws your way. Depending on the challenge, you could cruise through all four stages in a week. Or it could take several weeks to make it through a single step. It's okay if you're through a couple of steps on your journey and something happens in your path that causes you to take a step back to ensure you're back on track.

Now that you have your *Act As If...* steps in your back pocket and your mindset dialed in to learn such valuable information; you are ready to read on about things that will forever change the way you feel about yourself, about food, and fitness. Before reading on, take some time to write out any challenges you're facing, or anticipate facing that you could start to overcome with your *Act As If...* statement.

Write out your biggest Act As If... statement that speaks to you the most right now to get you moving towards your goal. Then, write out any actions you can take (do) that will move you into believing and achieving your goal:

Step 1: Act As If...

_____

_____

_____

_____

_____

Step 2: I will take action by doing...

_____

_____

_____

_____

_____

Step 3: I will believe in the following actions...

_____

_____

_____

_____

_____

Step 4: I will celebrate the following accomplishments by...

_____

_____

_____

_____

Finally, don't forget to celebrate your successes and milestones, whether big or small, whether it took a week to complete or three months. Success could be as simple as looking at and reading food labels when you never gave them a thought before. Keeping a positive growth mindset is a fantastic win to celebrate! Remember, this is where it all starts!

METHOD # 3:
Your Best Nutrition Plan Starts with Your BMR

You will gain the confidence and knowledge it takes to become your own working and efficient machine. You have what it takes to strengthen your mind and body to their fullest potential simply by taking over the wheel in the driver's seat and controlling the road to your health and fitness. Just be aware that this road will never be straight or smooth. You will experience right and left turns, bumps and rocks in the road, and you will learn the potholes to avoid. If you live in Pennsylvania, as I do, those roads are awful! But no matter what, you're still the driver and can willingly turn off the main road when you need to or turn on cruise control for a little while. Using the analogy to compare life to driving your car seems cliche, but it's so true.

You can only get so comfortable and so far using cruise control before you need to change your speed or change direction. Think about the new places you travel to. If you've never been there before, you will most likely need directions; if you have traveled the area frequently, you will no longer need guidance on how to get there. These upcoming chapters are so critical because they are your directions. It's okay to return to sections of this book down the road because it was less traveled (pun intended).

Sometimes we have setbacks, injuries, or sickness to work through. So instead of throwing in the towel, temporarily change your goal—this includes both activity and nutrition goals. I'll share a personal story to help paint that picture for you.

I had recently started my side career as a personal trainer while attending Penn State for my Kinesiology degree. Unfortunately, I had reinjured my knee, on which I had surgery for an anterior cruciate ligament (ACL) and meniscus repair. My current goal before reinjuring my knee was to build lean muscle through strength training. I was eating in such a way to support that goal—consuming additional calories and eating more nutritious carbohydrates and proteins than I would if I wasn't working towards this goal.

Ultimately, I had to get surgery again. Not only did that severely interfere with my activity level and fitness goal, but I needed to adjust my nutrition to reflect how much I had to scale back at the gym. I needed to switch my gears to *maintain* mode, which meant reducing the number of calories and how much of each macronutrient I was consuming. You may have scratched your head thinking, "I've heard that *m*-word before, but I don't know exactly what that is." We will get into what macronutrients are soon, but first, I must teach you about your basal metabolic rate (BMR), why it's essential to know, and how to figure it out.

Before you start any eating plan, knowing your basal metabolic rate, or BMR, is a must! Okay, so what's BMR, you ask? It's very different from your BMI (body mass index), so please don't get them confused!

Your basal metabolic rate is the number of calories your body requires at rest to complete life-sustaining (basal) functions like breathing and other organ functions.

Consuming under your BMR for long periods of time can cause your body the need to adapt—in other words—slow down to meet your basic functions. I see this many times with clients who are under-consuming calories and they struggle to lose weight or meet their fitness goals and they don't understand why. Eating less than what your body needs is not the answer to drop weight. When you slow down your metabolism, you prevent your body from functioning at its fullest potential. Regardless of your fitness and nutritional goals, if your BMR needs are not being met, your body will not be happy enough to make changes towards your goals.

Many of you reading this book probably never heard of BMR or know what it means. Why hasn't this significant nugget of knowledge ever been shared or addressed in all the diet plans out there? Almost every one of my clients had no clue what their BMR was or how to calculate it.

Think of the word basal. It makes me think of base, baseline, minimum, or where something starts. All of these words describe your first step in calculating how many calories you should be eating at a minimum. This knowledge is the first speck of light as you make your way out of the dark tunnel of mindless, unintentional eating, and there's no reason to ever feel in the dark about how much food your body requires again.

Now, let me tell you how to calculate this magnificent number! I've used a helpful and reliable website over the years to calculate BMR through calculator.net.

Calculate BMR

[Scan QR code] to calculate your BMR:

https://www.calculator.net/bmr-calculator.html

You can choose among the three formulas they provide to calculate your BMR. For example, if you know your body fat percentage, you may want to choose the formula that uses body fat. Under settings, it's the Katch-McArdle formula. BMR calculations are estimated formulas, but the formulas provided have been used in exercise science and kinesiology textbooks and are credited with giving close estimates of your caloric foundation.

Other available devices can calculate and provide body fat and BMR together, such as an InBody scan. The scan is similar to using the formula (with body fat) to figure out your BMR. Along with body fat and BMR, the scan will also break down intracellular and extracellular water—the amount of water inside and outside your cells in your body, respectively. It also provides you with segmental lean body mass weights and percentages. Again, what's the harm in knowing more about what's going on inside your body? Nothing at all, and it helps you in the long run by meeting your goals while seeing the changes along the way inside and outside of your body.

My anecdotal observation found that my clients who had taken photos, measurements, body fat, or InBody scan measurements had better adherence to whatever plan they were following. In addition, they reported an overall increase in happiness about their mood and lifestyle when working towards their goals.

Not knowing your lean body mass and water balance probably won't hinder a successful nutrition and fitness transformation. Still, I believe it is beneficial to know your body composition (body fat and muscle) at the very least. Knowing about your body and how your body functions is key to seeing a red flag before something wrong happens. Plus, it is misery if you rely only on your scale to measure success! You're missing out on many other changes that are taking place inside your body.

I had a client who I will call Greg. He was ready for a life change and willing to sacrifice whatever he needed to reach his goals. He had gone from almost entirely sedentary to working out thirty to forty minutes for four, sometimes five days each week. He also started tracking his calories, deciphering between what's a carbohydrate and what's not, and meeting protein and fat gram goals. The best thing about it is that he had all of the motivation in the world to make these changes; he just needed the tools—that's when he met with me.

Three to four weeks went by, and you could tell he was losing confidence in himself and me because he didn't really lose any weight. There are countless stories from people this happens to, and this is usually when people will throw in the towel. They may give up entirely or change to something super drastic and unhealthy. I get it; we live in a society where we want results now. If there were a pill you could take to look a certain way tomorrow, even though there could be many side effects, people would still be lined up to take it.

Luckily, I had done more than just take a starting weight from Greg at the beginning. We had other vital information like water balance, segmental lean body mass, and body fat. We did another analysis together, and, wouldn't you know, his body fat had gone down over 3 percent, and he had increased his lean muscle mass! Over the last month, changes had been taking place inside his body, yet it didn't look like he had made any progress at all on the scale. With all of the initial drastic changes he had made, you'd think weight would immediately start coming off.

I can't explain why sometimes weight drops off quickly for some and not for others, but I can tell you that the changes you make and the work you put into increasing your overall fitness level are worth it and working. Seeing those results were precisely what Greg needed to see to keep his spirits up and affirm that his hard work was paying off. Side note: Greg's weight significantly decreased just a week later, and he continued to change his body composition!

Don't rely solely on the scale—this one will be tough! If you don't have access to anything else that could provide body fat or lean muscle mass measurements, take pictures and use a tape measure for arms, legs, waist, and hips. Photographs are excellent at capturing those minor changes we miss day in and day out. You can be silly or serious, posed or unposed in your pictures—whatever it takes for you to capture your progress.

METHOD # 4:
Eating for Your Specific Fitness Goal

Regardless of your fitness goal, it all stems from your BMR. Depending on your chosen goal, you can decide how many additional calories you'll need above your BMR. Likewise, your macronutrient percentages for carbohydrates, protein, and fat will be determined by your fitness goal and what type of exercise you'd prefer to reach that goal.

Being intentional allows you to be more methodical with your eating, which gives you the most freedom with your food choices, leading to your success. I've been eating with intent for more than fifteen years. I promise you, eating does not feel like a chore. On the contrary, it gets easier as you learn and understand how foods work with your body and goals, not against them.

Fitness goals can change through different seasons of life, but conscientious eating should still be at the forefront, and hopefully, a trait of discipline that becomes a part of your lifestyle the more you practice it. Unfortunately, weight can creep on when you lose your intentions or change your fitness goal, but don't change your eating habits that go with it. Even if you don't have a fitness goal in mind, lose interest, or just take a break from whatever you're working toward, that's still a fitness goal—not actively working towards changing something but maintaining what you have at that current time.

There are goal-oriented subchapters outlining areas of fitness which include: weight or strength training, total body conditioning, cardiovascular fitness, and functional movement. Each goal subchapter will outline the importance, fuel source, and how to determine your macros to create your nutrition plan. In addition, my top food choices that I incorporate into my personal eating plan is in the back of the book in Appendix A: *Dani's Food Go-To's*.

You have the power to decide which foods will benefit you the most, so there is not specific foods that go along with each fitness goal. There are no *bad foods* or anything off-limits because this is not a food restriction nutrition plan. If you'd prefer to cut out particular foods or eat certain things sparingly, that's absolutely your choice. It's your nutrition plan for life, so let's live like it!

When you eat with macros in mind, you are learning to eat within limits. You can really have anything you want to eat, but fit those foods into a more structured plan. I'm a person who doesn't love a ton of rules, but let's be honest, if you have zero guidelines and everything's willy-nilly, it can spiral downhill without you even knowing you've lost all control. So, that's why I'm for structured guidelines. Stay within them, and you will be sure to succeed, but you can do whatever you want inside those guardrails—they are there, so you don't roll off the cliff.

With that being said, there is something worth saying about the quality of your food. It is possible to move towards your goals even when your food is not the healthiest, but I'm sure you will not feel your best. Highly processed foods usually lead to overindulgence and teach you absolutely nothing about the food itself, except how to open a package at lightning speed when it's time to eat!

I suggest reading through all of the different subchapters first, even if you know what specific fitness goal you desire. I've stuffed a lot of great information and relevant tips in each subchapter to help you understand the connection between fitness and nutrition. Look back to these subchapters as many times as you need. Your goals may change a couple of times throughout the year, depending on circumstance or an intentional change. No matter the reason for the change, I want you to feel equipped and confident in making all of those transitions by using this resource!

FITNESS GOAL:
Strength Or Weight Training

Why strength training is important: Strength training—or weight training—I use these words interchangeably, should be in your future in some shape or form to increase or preserve lean muscle. This fitness goal is so important that this should be on everyone's first or second goal priority list. Even if you're just looking to maintain or work on conditioning, we all lose muscle as we age!

Due to hormonal and muscular changes that happen as we age, we could lose from 3 to 8 percent per decade, starting as early as our thirties. So, guess what, folks? Whether you want to put any fitness goals on hold or just want to maintain what you've got, your lean muscle will decrease as you age, even if that is not your intent.

Having more lean muscle keeps metabolism running high, but muscle sarcopenia (muscle loss) happens as we age. As we lose muscle, body fat can creep up, and then our metabolism can slow down due to hormonal changes. It definitely has a snowball effect! So place strength training high on your priority list to preserve as much muscle as possible, keep a highly functioning metabolism, and keep body composition in check—remember, strong muscles protect and support your bones.

Fuel source: Carbohydrate is your body's preferred fuel source for weight and strength training (anaerobic training). Carbs are considered your body's most efficient fuel source because your body requires less oxygen to burn carbohydrates. For the purposes of this book, I'm not going to go into great detail about the mechanisms of how and why that happens at a cellular level but will keep it on a broader level for easier understanding.

Carbohydrates are not your enemy. Maybe more like your *frenemy* because there are so many unhealthy, sugar-loaded, highly processed carbohydrates out there that tend to become our only carbohydrate sources for the day. Yet, carbohydrates are vital in keeping your nervous system and brain functioning at optimal levels. We, as a society, just need to be filling up on the correct carbs—naturally derived or minimally processed.

When you ingest carbohydrate, it is either immediately used for energy or stored in muscles or the liver as glucose for later use. If we keep overeating carbs, don't use them for energy, and our glucose stores are filled, those extra calories are not needed and are potentially stored as fat. During exercise, your body will utilize glucose from those stores to provide steady blood glucose levels and prevent you from hypoglycemia or low blood sugar. It has shown to be an effective and optimal process to rely on liver and glycogen stores for energy and fuel for strength training.

When strength training is your focus, what you're essentially doing to your muscles is breaking them down. Tiny microscopic tears can happen within the muscle. Don't worry; you're not damaging your muscles in a bad way! These little tears lead to repairs and increased blood flow to your muscles, making them stronger and bigger. This process is called muscle hypertrophy or muscle growth.

This is the point at which protein comes into play. Protein is made up of smaller molecules called amino acids. You may have heard the words *amino acids* tossed out in conversation from someone at the gym or maybe read it on a recovery or post-workout drink label. Amino acids are proteins that make up muscles, tendons, and organs and regulate essential internal functions, such as your immune system.

Replenishing your muscles and body with protein has many benefits that make it worthwhile to seek out good quality protein for your nutrition plan. Protein will help build and repair muscles, leave you feeling more satiated, and can reduce appetite. You will find that most of my *go-to* protein sources are meat and dairy. I will also supplement with a whey protein powder. A side note when picking out a protein powder: If you're looking to increase protein intake, then most of the calories in your powder should be from protein. Pick a powder that is low in fat and carbohydrate. Personally, I like to buy my protein powder at a local supplement store. This way I can ask specific questions and express certain needs to someone who is able to provide guidance, rather than purchasing it online.

Since carbohydrates and proteins are our key players in any strength training program, they should be consumed in the most abundance. In addition, the right amount of healthy fats—foods high in polyunsaturated and monounsaturated fats—should be added to the plan for healthy brain function and heart health. These are named essential fatty acids for a reason and should not be avoided altogether. We can only get these essential fatty acids through our diet or supplements.

Fat Tip: Take note of your lower fat intake for strength training and building lean muscle. It's not because fat makes you fat (an abundance of calories does that!) Instead, proper carbohydrate and protein intake will allow your body to focus on muscle production from carbohydrates and protein synthesis from protein. In this case, fat is needed more for body function and support.

When picking fats to eat, they should be of importance. Think quality over quantity for this one! There are essential fats that are needed because they are crucial for some pretty big things that happen inside your body, and our bodies do not produce these types of fats.

Include dietary fats such as Omega-3 and Omega-6 fatty acids, which are polyunsaturated fats and monounsaturated fats. Examples of food high in these essential fatty acids are mackerel, salmon, flax seeds, chia seeds, walnuts, egg yolks, soybeans, and tofu. Fats also support cell membrane structure and function, provide insulation, regulate temperature, and metabolize fat-soluble vitamins such as A, D, E, and K. These vitamins require fat to be absorbed properly and used in the body, something you definitely don't want to miss out on.

If you follow the recommendations from the table below, the percentages should allow for enough carbohydrates to readily use and store for later use in the muscles and liver. Optimal protein recommendations for strength training can range from 0.8 to 1.2 grams consumed per pound of body weight. I prefer to use total percentages when setting up my eating plans, so by setting your intake at 35 to 40 percent, most people would easily be in the recommended range.

If your protein percentage recommendation from Table 1 is not within 0.8 to 1.2 grams per pound of body weight, you can increase or decrease your protein percentage to land you somewhere within that range. For example, if you multiply your body weight by 0.8 and 1.2 and your calculated protein grams are not in between the two numbers, then increase or decrease your protein grams to fall within that range. Likewise, you can split the difference between your carbohydrate and fat percentages. This could potentially happen if you're significantly over or underweight.

Table 1. Macronutrient Percentages for Weight Training

Carbohydrate Needs	40-50% of total calories
Protein Needs	35-40% of total calories
Fat Needs	15-20% of total calories

I'll use a female weighing 160 pounds with a BMR of 1422 calories (Height, weight, age, and gender all played a factor in figuring out her BMR using the website I shared with you). Her goal is to lose weight while building lean muscle. Her BMR was used in the example in the first row using Table 1.1.

CONVERSION TIP!
When converting protein, carbohydrate, and fat calories into grams: Divide calories by 4 when converting carbohydrates and protein to grams;Divide calories by 9 when converting fat to grams.

*Note, you can increase your carbs up to 50% and drop the percentages for protein and fat, so the total equals 100% if you feel that your energy needs are not being met at the other percentages and vice versa. Listen to your body; you will feel what it needs.

*Round calories to the nearest one. Replace your own BMR in place of 1422 when doing calculations for yourself.

Macro Break-Down Equation:

(BMR) X (macro %) = calories needed and gram conversion.

Table 1.1 Macronutrient Calculations for Calories & Grams

Macronutrient	Macro %	BMR x % = calories	Calories ÷ 4 or 9 = Grams
Example	*40%*	*1422 x 0.40 = 569*	*569 ÷ 4 = 142*
Carbohydrate	40%	x 0.40 =	÷ 4 =
Carbohydrate	45%	x 0.45 =	÷ 4 =
Carbohydrate	50%	x 0.50 =	÷ 4 =
Protein	35%	x 0.35 =	÷ 4 =
Protein	40%	x 0.40 =	÷ 4 =
Fat	15%	x 0.15 =	÷ 9 =
Fat	20%	x 0.20 =	÷ 9 =

Determining daily caloric intakes: Now, it's time to determine how many additional calories you need above your BMR, which will ultimately depend on your goal. Remember, these are estimates, and you may need to increase or decrease your caloric intake to match your needs inside or outside these ranges to feel your best and get the results you desire.

If you want to lose weight while building lean muscle: Your goal is to create a deficit through your activity, not by starving yourself or dropping your calories below your BMR. The key is to drop weight and body fat while still having enough energy to power through workouts. It is possible to build lean muscle while keeping calories slightly above your BMR. Muscle growth may not occur as quickly as adding more calories for growth, but if dropping body fat is most important to you, then that should be your focus. If you're doing the right workouts for building lean muscle, even on a lower-calorie nutrition plan, you will benefit from decreasing body fat and building lean muscle.

Increase calories above your BMR from 200 to 500 calories. If workouts and daily activities seem strenuous, you may feel better adding closer to 500 calories. But our lives are ever-changing, so your eating should change to match your life. For example, if you know you're not working out as much or are more sedentary one week, tweak your calories to the lower end of 200. It is okay for your calories to fluctuate up or down within your range daily or weekly, depending on days off from the gym.

If you want to maintain weight and lean muscle: Your goal is to match your calories in with your calories out. Your *total daily energy expenditure* (TDEE) is the total energy a person uses daily, but this can be hard to figure out. Aside from varying day-to-day, other estimated measures such as activity level, BMR, and thermic effect of food affect your TDEE. You can use devices like watches and other wearable monitors that track calories you burned during your workouts. If you do not track calories by a device you wear, you can use the TDEE calculator.

You will be able to pick the type and amount of exercise you do. If using the calculator, you will want to take notice of the calculated number, and how much higher it is above your BMR. That will give you a ballpark of your weekly calorie burn. Don't forget that formulas and devices used to track calories are estimations. If you feel like you are eating way under what you are burning, then increase your calories. If you think that the expenditure estimates are over what you burn each day, then decrease calories a little each day. This is all about fine-tuning! Since these are estimates, and it isn't easy to know if you are burning a couple hundred calories over or under the calculated TDEE, you should continually monitor and adjust calorie intake based on your progress and intuitions.

[Scan the QR code] to calculate your TDEE:

Calculate TDEE

If you want to gain weight and build lean muscle: The overall goal of weight gain should not just be eating everything in sight to have a significant increase in body fat—though gaining weight and eating more might be exciting. The purpose is to fuel your precious machine while building lean muscle tissue and keeping your body fat in check. Make sure your fitness goal of building lean muscle reflects your effort and workouts. If you overeat and don't put those calories to good use through a strength training program, you will be left with a softer, more plump figure rather than a thicker, more muscular look.

Going off of your BMR, add an additional 1000 to 1500 calories. To replace those calories used, you may also need to add extra calories to replace those burned during workouts, depending on the duration and intensity of the activity. Tracking your average calories burned can help with this. For example, if you have a super strenuous job and tend to burn many calories during the day, plus you're weight training most days of the week and trying to gain weight, I would start at the highest level of calories and adjust from there. So how do you know if you're adding too many calories that could have a negative impact? First, you figure out your upper limit.

Our bodies have an upper limit caloric intake, which we fully metabolize and utilize the nutrients we consume. Similarly, our BMR is our lower limit, which we shouldn't go below for optimal health. So it makes sense that every person's upper limit would be different, just like their lower limit differs. Don't just pull a number out of the air because you heard of some athlete eating thousands and thousands of calories. Instead, take the time to calculate your upper limit to get the maximum absorption from food, so you're not just eating for the sake of eating that adds unwanted weight gain.

Your upper caloric limit is typically 2.5 times your BMR. To calculate this, you would multiply your BMR by 2.5. Let's use the BMR from above of 1422 in the sample calculation below:

Upper Caloric Limit → 1422 x 2.5 = 3,555 calories

Types of Exercises or Workouts that Fall Under Strength/Weight Training:

1. Bodybuilding
2. Off-season team sports to increase mass
3. Strength & conditioning
4. Recreational lifter

FITNESS GOAL:
Total Body Conditioning

Why total body conditioning is important: Personally, I prefer this training style and macro percentages for my training most of the year. The other part of the year my focus will be dedicated solely to strength training. Total body conditioning (TBC) includes components of strength training, HIIT (high-intensity interval training), muscular endurance, and functional training/movements. This training goal is perfect for anyone seeking their inner athlete who desires to feel stronger, more conditioned, and wants to achieve a well-rounded fitness level.

A TBC workout can vary in time and intensity. Usually, if your intensity is higher, the duration of your workout is shorter. Endurance workouts or low- to moderate-intensity exercises are typically longer in duration. However, the more conditioned you become, your intensity or duration can increase in a single bout of exercise—or both can increase!

When I competed in 2018 and in 2022 in bodybuilding in the figure division, I had a total body conditioning focus in between the two competitions, which kept me lean and toned. I switched my goal to strength training to gain more muscle several months before my competition before switching back to conditioning in preparation for my show.

I still gained muscle while in my TBC focus, but by really centering my training and eating around strength training made all the difference. I had about four months to focus on putting on as much muscle as I could, so not only did my training differ, but my nutrition had to follow suit. I set up my macro percentages, aiming to gain muscle and gain some weight during that time while keeping my body fat around what it was before I started.

In that time, I gained seven pounds and had only put on half a percent of body fat by following the strength training nutrition plan I laid out earlier in this chapter. The extra weight accounted for an increase in overall total body water, muscle, and body fat. I wanted to maintain the muscle I had gained but needed a leaner, more conditioned look while preserving muscle—time to switch gears and change my focus back to total body conditioning!

The macro percentages will change slightly, but as with any nutritional plan, we start with our BMR. The most significant change you will see is increased fats and decreased carbohydrates. With TBC, your primary fuel source isn't as straightforward as strength training, which primarily relies on carbohydrates. Both energy systems can be utilized— anaerobic and aerobic, or without oxygen and with oxygen; so fuel comes from carbohydrates and fats, respectively. Your nutritional plan will be flexible with carbohydrate and fat percentages. Depending on the style or emphasis of training you lean towards, you can choose the high end of the recommended fat range with a lower carbohydrate range for more aerobic conditioning, or choose a higher range for carbohydrate and lower range for fat for more anaerobic conditioning. If your training is split, you can set your ranges so they are closer together.

Fuel source: To fuel your workout, you will utilize carbohydrates and fats with a little more emphasis on carbohydrates over fat. Protein will be vital for recovery, muscle repair, and cell signaling. We want to make sure that we use the good carbohydrates and fats available in our bodies as fuel, rather than using protein as a fuel source. If protein is used as a fuel supply, you could experience muscle catabolism—the breakdown of skeletal muscle to use as fuel. It's very inefficient for your body to use protein as fuel, but it will do what it needs to if you're not giving yourself adequate calories and macronutrients to match your workout requirements.

From reading about carbohydrates in the subchapter before, we know that our bodies utilize carbs for high-intensity exercise that doesn't require oxygen (anaerobic), so carbs are best used for weight training. Carbs also aid in the metabolism of fat. Therefore, to effectively burn fat, your body must first break down a certain amount of carbs before burning fat, or else it may not burn fat in the most effective way. Lastly, the fewer carbohydrates we eat, the lower our glycogen stores are from which we pull energy. So eating the right amount of carbohydrates really does matter in order for our bodies to produce the most effective workout with maximum effort.

Now, let's move on to fat as a fuel source. We all have an abundance of body fat to use as fuel. Yes, even those lean machines who walk around the gym with very low body fat still have enough fat to fuel workouts. Besides the fat we can see and grab, we have fat within our muscles and around our organs to help protect them.

Just as carbohydrates aid in maximizing fat burning, the body uses fat to help access stored glycogen. Utilizing and burning fat is more of a process than using carbohydrates (even though fat is readily available) and requires oxygen (aerobic). Fat is slow to digest, so eating a bunch of fat before a workout isn't a great idea. After eating fat, it also needs time to be broken down and transported to muscles.

We do not have an abundance of body fat from eating too much fat; we accumulate an abundance of fat from eating too many calories, decreasing exercise that utilizes and burns carbohydrates and fat, and lack of discipline. Therefore, it's okay to eat high-fat foods like avocados, egg yolks, almonds, and other nuts and seeds.

Our bodies burn fat during low- to moderate-intensity exercise but require a great deal of oxygen. The oxygen needed is usually at or below 65 percent of your aerobic capacity or 50 to 70 percent of your maximum heart rate. So, when referring to the amount of intensity in your moderate state—your breathing quickens, but you should still be able to speak three to five words per breath, and you will usually start to sweat after about ten minutes.

High-intensity exercise falls in the range of 70 to 85 percent of your maximum heart rate. During this type of vigorous activity, your breathing is deep and rapid. After a few minutes of the exercise, you typically begin to sweat and may be able to say only a few words in between breaths.

To figure out your maximum heart rate, or MHR, you simply take your age and subtract it from 220. Like most things pertaining to our bodies, this calculation is an estimation and can vary from person to person by ten to twenty beats. Once you know your MHR, you can determine your low- to moderate- to high-intensity ranges by multiplying MHR by 0.5, 0.7, and 0.85, respectively. I'll talk more about max heart rate and percentages in the cardiovascular endurance subchapter, but I wanted to make you aware of how your intensities would look and feel.

To calculate Maximum Heart Rate (MHR): 220 - age = MHR

Ultimately, we want our metabolism to run as efficiently as possible so we feel and look our best. If your fitness goal is to do total body conditioning, utilizing both anaerobic (without oxygen) and aerobic (with oxygen) energy pathways, then eating the proper proportion of macros should reflect that.

In Table 2, you will see that the percentage of carbohydrates for total body conditioning does not need to be as high as the percentage required for weight training because you will not depend on exercise that relies mainly on carbohydrates for fuel. Fats have been increased to make up for the decrease in total carbohydrates, and protein has stayed relatively the same to aid in muscle recovery, fluid balance, cell signaling, and other critical hormonal functions in the body.

Table 2. Calculating Your Macros for Total Body Conditioning

Carbohydrate Needs	35-40% of total calories
Protein Needs	35% of total calories
Fat Needs	25-30% of total calories

Conversion Tip!
When converting protein, carbohydrate, and fat calories into grams: Divide calories by 4 when converting carbohydrates and protein to grams; Divide calories by 9 when converting fat to grams.

To determine your calorie needs for each macronutrient category, first, find your BMR. Instructions for the best way to calculate your BMR can be found in Method 3 on page 36. First, let's use the example of a female with a BMR of 1422.

*Calories are rounded to the nearest whole calorie. Place your own BMR in place of the example 1422 when doing calculations for yourself.

Macro Break-Down Equation:
(BMR) X (macro %) = calories needed
Table 2.1 Macronutrient Calculations for Calories & Grams

Macronutrient	Macro %	BMR x % = calories	Calories ÷ 4 or 9 = Grams
Example	*35%*	*1422 x 0.35 = 498*	*498 ÷ 4 = 125*
Carbohydrate	35%	x 0.35 =	÷ 4 =
Carbohydrate	40%	x 0.40 =	÷ 4 =
Protein	35%	x 0.35 =	÷ 4 =
Fat	20%	x 0.20 =	÷ 9 =
Fat	25%	x 0.25 =	÷ 9 =

Determining daily caloric intakes: Now, it's time to determine how many additional calories you need above your BMR, which will ultimately depend on your goal. Remember, these are estimates, and you may need to increase or decrease your caloric intake to match your needs inside or outside these ranges to feel your best and get the results you desire.

If you want to lose weight: Remember that your goal is to create a deficit through your activity, not by starving yourself or dropping your calories below your BMR (basal metabolic rate). You can start by adding 200 to 400 calories to your calculated BMR. It's okay to change your calorie range depending on your day and whether you work out or not. Taking a day off from a workout is no problem; you can adjust your caloric intake for the day to the lower end of your range above your BMR that

61

day. Or maybe you hit the gym hard almost every day and had some great sweat sessions; you might feel more hungry and need the additional calories each day.

If you want to maintain weight: This daily caloric intake is more for muscle maintenance, but muscle growth can occur in this dietary fitness goal as well. Total body conditioning has endless ways and techniques to put new strains and stresses on muscles for growth to occur, as well as burning extra calories overall in a single workout.

To maintain your weight, your goal should be to match your calories in and out. Logging or tracking your food for a minimum of three days, or ideally for seven days, will give you the best snapshot of your average daily caloric intake. You can also use a TDEE calculator to help provide you with an estimate. Refer back to page ___to use the QR code for the TDEE calculator.

If your goal is to increase lean muscle mass: You can start by adding in an additional 300 to 600 calories daily, or every other day, in addition to the calories you would need to match your calories in/calories out (maintenance weight). A healthy amount of weight to put on should be between half a pound to one-and-a-half pounds per month. You do not want to carelessly add weight to your figure, so gaining weight every week will put you at a higher chance of adding unwanted body fat along with your muscle.

Types of Exercises or Workouts that Fall Under Total Body Conditioning:

1. Cross-training or Circuit training
2. Kettlebell training

3. Most group fitness classes—circuit training, TRX, HIIT classes, boot camps, interval, kickboxing, and conditioning
4. Athletic conditioning
5. Cross-fit
6. Bodyweight training—calisthenics, push-ups, pull-ups, sit-ups, and other functional movements
7. Equipment training—battle ropes, sled, medicine balls, sand balls, boxes (for box jumps), hurdles, exercise bands, Jacob's ladder, and ladder (foot drills)

FITNESS GOAL:
Cardiovascular Fitness

Why it's important: Working on and improving your cardiovascular fitness increases the efficiency of your heart, lungs, and blood vessels. In addition, it can improve circulation, making it easier to pump blood through your body. If you're a runner or other endurance athlete, maybe these things are secondary interests compared to increasing your race performance. Either way, you get the benefit of decreased heart disease.

I don't enjoy doing cardio by myself. You'll never hear me say, "I'm going for a run," just because I want to get my heart pumping. However, I am a decent runner supporter. If someone asks me to go for a run, a bike ride, or anything in a group setting, I will do it. I definitely prefer cardiovascular group fitness classes to improve my cardiovascular fitness. I do teach spin, after all, and I love it!

There are several significant numbers to learn and know if your primary fitness goal is to improve cardiovascular fitness. Unlike using how heavy your weights are and total exercise volume as a benchmark for progress, you need to focus on heart rate, VO2-max, and time as indicators.

After calculating your maximum heart rate (220 - Age = MHR), you can use MHR to know what *zones* you're essentially training in. The maximum heart rate calculation is a close estimation. Your efficiency and conditioning can affect your max heart rate cardiovascular exercise calculations.

You might be wondering what VO2-max is? Your VO2-max is your maximal aerobic capacity or maximal oxygen uptake. In other words, VO2-max measures the amount or volume of oxygen an individual can utilize in one minute. For the general population or recreational fitness enthusiasts, figuring this out may not be of interest to you. Still, if you want to figure it out, you can use the QR code below to calculate your VO2-max.

Calculate VO2-Max

[Scan QR Code] to calculate VO2-Max

https://www.omnicalculator.com/sports/vo2-max

Time is a great way to gauge progress when performing cardiovascular exercise, and it's easy to do! Let's just say you start by running a 15-minute mile. Then, as you keep training over the weeks, you should become more efficient at running not only in your breathing but also in your conditioning as well, and before you know it, you are running 13-minute, 12-minute, and then 10-minute miles.

You can go the other way, too, to track progress or know if you are becoming faster and stronger by setting a specific time and monitoring how far you can go. For example, you perform thirty minutes of cardio on the elliptical or treadmill every day. Even though your time stays the same, the distance can vary each time depending on your effort output. You can track and try to beat your distance each day or use the total mileage for the week.

There is a game on the rower at the gym I introduced to my clients because many people, like myself, don't enjoy doing cardio solo. So, instead of dreading the monotonous thought of cardio, you can spice it up with a game. I like it because you do have to put forth the effort, unlike placing yourself in front of a TV for a distraction where you can expend little to no effort.

It's called the *Fish Game*. It counts down from four minutes, and the point of the game is to eat as many fish as you can as you row. Large fish are sixty points, and small fish are thirty points. However, as the fish are swimming by the screen, so are sharks that can eat your fish and eat you! If you are eaten, you lose forty-five points, disappear for a second or two, then you come back and resume the game.

I often play this game, and let me tell you, after four minutes on the rower, my heart is pounding, and sweat is beading on my face and body. The extrinsic motivator is to beat your high score from the time before. The game also tracks the distance you row in meters, which is what I look at. Each time I hop on to play the Fish Game, it will give me the same four minutes. The computerized shark and fish patterns change up a bit, but I can start to guess where they will go next. The distance my clients or I travel depends totally on the person rowing. Covering more distance, in the same amount of time, shouts, "Progress!" You were able to cover more ground and put out more effort in the same amount of time given.

My friends, the progress and success you experience on the rower is worth cheering about. You can complete several rounds in a row and compare distances for each of the rounds. Which round did you go the furthest? Was it at the beginning while you were fresh, or was during your last round to push past your other distances? It's amazing to see how far we can truly push when we are distracted with competition. Check for games on other pieces of exercise equipment too! You can also create your own games by setting timers, adding intervals, and different fun ways to keep yourself moving and challenged.

Fuel source: Fat is optimal for fueling low- to moderate-intensity exercise. Fat fuels those longer-duration workouts, sparing your glycogen stores (from carbohydrates). Typically, when the duration of our exercise becomes longer, our intensity decreases, and we can utilize fat for fuel. At low- to moderate-intensity exercise, you can rely on fat for fuel and use stored muscle and liver glycogen at a slow rate, delaying fatigue and prolonging activity.

Speaking of prolonged activity, what about training for longer runs or bike rides? Again, carbohydrates can aid in energy production for times your body needs it—for example, half marathons and full marathons. In addition, there's a method that can help called carb-loading or carb cycling.

Carb-Loading & Carb Cycling

In a nutshell, carb cycling and loading is when you manipulate your carbohydrate intake by increasing or decreasing the amount throughout the week instead of keeping carbs at a target percent, as I've taught you. Your overall caloric intake doesn't have to increase, but it can. If your calories stay the same, you will decrease the amount of fat when you increase carbs, but protein stays steady.

Carb-Loading: The benefit of increasing carbohydrates before a long exercise bout (over two hours) is to increase the amount of glycogen stored in the liver and muscles. Proper carb-loading should be done over two days, so one large spaghetti meal the day before your race isn't going to cut it. Instead, strategic preparation and planning are needed to execute a carb-load correctly, so you get the full benefit on race day.

Seven days before your race day, you should do an intense and vigorous workout to deplete your carbs. You were probably nodding along reading that because you know high-intensity workouts require carbs. Then for several days, you want to eat a lower-carb diet with similar percentages to those laid out for you in Table 3. However, you could even drop carbs by as much as 20 percent. Think of this process as a see-saw: protein is steady in the middle (as your base), and if carbs go down, fats must go up. So your workouts should be light to moderate. Since you're dropping the percentage of carbohydrates, they must go somewhere, so your total percentage intake equals one hundred percent. Whatever you take away from carbs, you can add it to your fat percentage.

Two days prior to race day, carbs should increase from 70 to 75 percent, and the remaining 25 to 30 percent should come mainly from protein. Imagine another see-saw on which the fats plummet to the ground and carbohydrates soar up to the sky. Overall work volume should dramatically decrease as well.

Research has shown that loading your carbohydrates this way has a positive increase in muscle and liver glycogen stores. An increase in storage means more energy for a longer period of time. And where there are carbs, there is water. Retaining more water on race day isn't a bad thing; it can actually help prevent dehydration. That's why carb-loading works well with long endurance events.

Carb-Cycling: Carb cycling comes from the same idea and has been adopted as a way of eating for athletes, recreational exercisers, and even for the average Joe Shmoe. From a health point of view, studies suggest that carb cycling may improve insulin sensitivity and weight loss. From a performance and aesthetic perspective, this way of eating, unlike long-term low-carb eating, will provide enough energy for low-, medium- or high-intensity workouts, decreases body fat, and prevents the feeling of brain fog.

The popularity of carb cycling gained much traction in the bodybuilding world. I will use carb cycling in phases as a part of my training leading up to my show. I know this might be another head-scratcher moment. You just learned that your body prefers carbohydrates as fuel during strenuous exercise, so how can low-carb mixed with high-carb eating be beneficial? I can't give you reasons why others do it, but I can tell you why I like incorporating it into my regimen and the advantages I've seen and felt.

Switching to carb cycling for periods of time has helped my body utilize all of the carbohydrates I eat on high-carb day for energy, and fully emptying my glycogen stores through my low-carb days. I'm not dragging with low energy because I add in a high-carb day when I feel like my carbs are depleted, and I can reap the benefits of regulated insulin levels, gain lean muscle, and keep a lean figure all at the same time. I would recommend carb cycling for people who like variations in their diet and want to plan. It's also good for people who prefer to eat carbohydrates dispersed throughout the week.

A typical carb cycling schedule follows the same cycling schedule, but how often you add in high carb days can differ week to week and person to person. I will start with two or three low-carb days, followed by one high-carb day, and carry out that eating pattern weekly. Another way of setting up a carb cycling schedule would be to pick specific days of the week to implement a high-carb day. For example, I have picked Wednesday and Sunday to eat high carbs to recharge, and the remaining days would be low-carb eating that week. To go one step further, I would schedule my heaviest or highest volume of training around my high-carb days because those are the days I'll need high carbohydrates the most and to feel my best.

So, if this is something you'd like to implement while you're working towards any of your fitness goals, I suggest following your nutritional plan given for your particular fitness goal for the first four to six weeks before jumping into carb cycling. Having your head wrapped around a base nutrition plan first will help you understand the differences between carbohydrates, proteins, and fats and will help you master the art of carb cycling.

Table 3. Calculating Your Macros for Cardiovascular Endurance

Carbohydrate Needs	30-35% of total calories
Protein Needs	30-35% of total calories
Fat Needs	30-40% of total calories

Conversion Tip!

When converting protein, carbohydrate, and fat calories into grams: Divide calories by 4 when converting carbohydrates and protein to grams; Divide calories by 9 when converting fat to grams.

To determine your calorie needs for each macronutrient category, find your BMR. Instructions for the best way to calculate your BMR can be found in Method 3 on page 36.

*Calories are rounded to the nearest whole calorie. Put your own BMR in place of 1422 when doing your own calculations.

Macro Break-Down Equation:
(BMR) X (macro %) = calories needed
Table 3.1 Macronutrient Calculations for Calories & Grams

(Macro Percentages from Table 3)

Macronutrient	Macro %	BMR x % = calories	Calories ÷ 4 or 9 = Grams
Example	*30%*	*1422 x 0.30 = 427*	*427 ÷ 4 = 107*
Carbohydrate	30%	x 0.30 =	÷ 4 =
Carbohydrate	35%	x 0.35 =	÷ 4 =
Protein	30%	x 0.30 =	÷ 4 =
Protein	35%	x 0.35 =	÷ 4 =
Fat	30%	x 0.30 =	÷ 9 =
Fat	35%	x 0.35 =	÷ 9 =
Fat	40%	x 0.40 =	÷ 9 =

Table 3.2 Calculating Your Macros for Carb Cycling

High Carb Day	
Carbohydrate Needs	60-70% of total calories
Protein Needs	25-35% of total calories
Fat Needs	5-10% of total calories
Low Carb Day	
Carbohydrate Needs	10-20% of total calories
Protein Needs	30-35% of total calories
Fat Needs	45-60% of total calories

Table 3.3 Macronutrient Calculations for Calories & Grams (Macro Percentages from Table 3.2)

High Carb Day			
Macronutrient	**Macro %**	**BMR x % = calories**	**Calories ÷ 4 or 9 = Grams**
Example	*60%*	*1422 x 0.60 = 853*	*853 ÷ 4 = 213*
Carbohydrate	60%	x 0.60 =	÷ 4 =
Carbohydrate	65%	x 0.65 =	÷ 4 =
Carbohydrate	70%	x 0.70 =	÷ 4 =
Protein	25%	x 0.25 =	÷ 4 =
Protein	30%	x 0.30 =	÷ 4 =
Protein	35%	x 0.35 =	÷ 4 =
Fat	5%	x 0.05 =	÷ 9 =
Fat	10%	x 0.10 =	÷ 9 =

Table 3.4 Macronutrient Calculations for Calories & Grams (Macro Percentages from Table 3.2)

Low Carb Day			
Macronutrient	**Macro %**	**BMR x % = calories**	**Calories ÷ 4 or 9 = Grams**
Example	*10%*	*1422 x 0.10 = 142*	*142 ÷ 4 = 36*
Carbohydrate	10%	x 0.10 =	÷ 4 =
Carbohydrate	15%	x 0.15 =	÷ 4 =
Carbohydrate	20%	x 0.20 =	÷ 4 =
Protein	30%	x 0.30 =	÷ 4 =
Protein	35%	x 0.35 =	÷ 4 =
Fat	45%	x 0.45 =	÷ 9 =
Fat	50%	x 0.50 =	÷ 9 =
Fat	55%	x 0.55 =	÷ 9 =
Fat	60%	x 0.60 =	÷ 9 =

Determining daily caloric intakes: Now, it's time to determine how many additional calories you need above your BMR, which will ultimately depend on your goal. Remember, these are estimates, and you may need to increase or decrease your caloric intake to match your needs inside or outside these ranges to feel your best and get the results you desire.

If you want to lose weight: Start by calculating your BMR and setting your macros to the recommended ranges for this fitness goal. How high above your BMR you can set your calories for weight loss will depend on the frequency and duration of your cardiovascular exercise.

My insider tip that will help you here is that you have to burn about 3500 calories to lose a pound. So, if your goal is to lose one pound per week, you would have to burn an additional 500 calories per day if you set your calories close to your BMR. It would be best if you did not dip below your BMR to create a bigger deficit or compensate for calories not burned during the day. Burning an extra 500 calories per day doesn't just have to come from exercise alone.

Think about the activity you do during the day that burns calories. For example, if you have a pretty sedentary work life and your daily living is low-key, it would probably benefit you to workout most days of the week. But if you have a demanding job and a moderately active lifestyle, skipping a workout or two during the week wouldn't affect your overall progress. To ballpark your daily expenditure, refer to Method 3 on page 51 to calculate your TDEE (total daily energy expenditure).

If you are sedentary, you could start by setting your calorie goal 100 to 200 calories above your BMR. Then, you can gradually increase your daily calories by 100 to 200 the more active you are. To lose weight for this fitness goal, you typically wouldn't need to increase your additional calories by more than 600 to 800 above your BMR.

Weight loss tip: If you are doing cardio strictly for weight loss, I suggest adding strength training to your fitness regimen for several reasons. Cardio burns fat, but cardio does not shape or tone your body or muscles. Both men and women have come to me for help after losing weight by primarily doing cardio because they were unhappy with their lack of muscle tone and shape. I also found that those who focused on cardio for weight loss took a lot longer to achieve their weight loss goal than those who incorporated strength training and cardio in their exercise program.

Strength training can increase the number of calories you burn at rest for twenty-four hours after exercise. The increased metabolic burn can vary from person to person, but, collectively determined, there was an overall increase in the calories burned at rest after strength training. In contrast, after a cardio session, whatever calories were burned during that session are just that—calories burned—and seemed to have no effect on the rate at which you burn calories for the rest of the 24-hour period.

The question that arises in this section is what nutrition plan should you follow if you start incorporating strength training? Even if you start strength training two days per week and the rest of the days are cardio, follow the strength training nutrition program I've laid out for you. Then, you can integrate more strength training days into your exercise plan as you see fit with your progress.

If you want to maintain weight & increase stamina & endurance: Play around with the macro percentages given within this subchapter. The key thing is that you are eating properly. Proper eating enables you to push through and increase intensity over time to see and feel a difference in your cardiovascular endurance.

If you increase the duration of your exercise and don't want to lose weight, make sure you match your calorie needs and expenditure.

That will most likely mean increasing calories. Even when you increase your calories, your macro percentages stay as they are. If you reached your desired weight goal and are already eating 400 calories over your BMR, you can add in an additional 50 to 100 calories a day until you can maintain. For example, you may find to sustain your weight at your current exercise regimen, you need to eat an additional 550 calories over your BMR daily. Those extra calories are distributed between your carbohydrates, protein, and fats based on the percentages you are following.

Types of Exercises or Workouts that Fall Under Cardiovascular Fitness:

1. Walking, jogging, running
2. Elliptical, cross-trainers, rowing, or other pieces of cardio equipment
3. Biking, skating, skateboarding
4. Hiking
5. Dancing
6. Group fitness classes—Zumba, POUND, step, spin, cardio kickboxing, shadow boxing, and other aerobic-based classes

FITNESS GOAL:
Functional Movement & Flexibility (A good starting point for non-exercisers!)

Why functional movement and flexibility are important: Performing daily tasks with minimal risk of injury to yourself is an essential part of your well-being and living your best life. Being capable and comfortable in your own skin should be at the top of everyone's list. For example, how easy is it to bend over and tie your shoes, reach and lift objects, or twist your core?

If you've been reading up to this point, I hope I have enticed you to seek out some avenues of fitness that you never thought about doing or want to know more about. It is never too late to start working on your nutrition and fitness. Start with a simple commitment to doing something every week. Go check out a local gym, join a friend in their workout, ask your accountability partner to meet for a workout session, or search up exercises that interest you on the internet. These days you can get full workout plans and videos of entire workouts for just about every need. You are well equipped with your Act As If. . . plan. I expect you to use it on yourself and share your knowledge with others to spread positivity and make a difference in other people's lives.

I had a client—I'll call her Sheila. She had never touched a weight, been in a gym, or really exercised in her life before we met. She was aggravated and disappointed with the way she looked. She came to me to begin her journey with better nutrition. I could see she was uncomfortable in her own skin, wearing layers of clothing to hide the mess she felt she had made of herself.

She wasn't a mess at all. On the contrary, she was desperate to get back to her old self but was definitely left with scars of defeat from the ten-plus diets she'd tried in the past—each had left her carrying more weight than before she dieted.

From the start, she had no interest in joining a gym. We chatted about what she did for a living, and the limited time she had outside of family time, work, and some social clubs she's associated with, and I found she really did have a tight but regimented schedule. Sheila's nutrition was spiraling out of control, but my girl, Sheila, liked her structure.

Sheila expressed that she started having pain in places she'd never experienced before, and it was affecting the things she enjoyed doing, like gardening around the house and simple tasks like going up and down the stairs. I knew the extra weight she was carrying wasn't helping with any of those issues, but I think her diet was contributing to inflammation discomfort.

First, we started with obstacles that could potentially get in the way of her success. I'm not going to lie, there were several obstacles written out, and she didn't feel confident about overcoming them. Her second step was to start with an Act As If. . . goal. Then she started the nutrition plan that I outlined in this subchapter.

Let's fast forward to the end of the old Sheila. We had check-ins over several months to keep her accountable and on track. I didn't start her off right away with exercise because I knew it would be too much. So if you don't start that way either, that's okay. After about three weeks of concentrating on her nutrition, I gave Sheila functional movement exercises—about fifteen minutes worth—to incorporate every day. She then wanted to incorporate forty-five to sixty-minute power walks on Saturdays and Sundays since the pain she had been experiencing was completely gone! She switched her nutrition plan to TBC after discovering that she loved activity and exercises in intervals and gained a new perspective of fitness and confidence in herself.

I love client stories like Sheila's. Time and time again, she went from hopeful to hopeless, doubting herself more and more every time a diet failed her. But, learning to appreciate food for what it is and what it can do for your body can make an everlasting impact. It's not about the quick fixes; it's about taking the step in the right direction, listening to your body, and tuning out the social pressures to set your mind right!

Fuel source: A combination of carbohydrates and fat will be your fuel source. Protein is still needed in a reasonable amount in any nutrition plan, even if you're not working out or performing light activity. This nutrition plan has a good balance of carbohydrates and fats, with protein coming in somewhat lower than in other plans that have higher amounts of physical activity.

I often see protein tossed to the side by individuals who think it's only for building muscle. Eating more protein will not pack muscle onto your body—I wish! You need to put in the work for muscle growth to occur. From reading all the excellent information about protein, carbohydrates, and fats in the previous subchapters, you are already in the know—you just need to balance them out to match your goal.

Table 4

Calculating Your Macros for *Functional Movement & Flexibility*

Carbohydrate Needs	35-40% of total calories
Protein Needs	25% of total calories
Fat Needs	35-40% of total calories

Conversion Tip!
When converting protein, carbohydrate, and fat calories into grams: Divide calories by 4 when converting carbohydrates and protein to grams; Divide calories by 9 when converting fat to grams.

To determine your calorie needs for each macronutrient category, first find your BMR. Instructions for the best way to calculate your BMR can be found in Method 3 on page 36.

Calories are rounded to the nearest whole calorie. Place your own BMR in place of 1422 when doing your calculations.

Macro Break-Down Equation:

(BMR) X (macro %) = calories needed

Table 4.1 Macronutrient Calculations for Calories & Grams

Macronutrient	Macro %	BMR x % = calories	Calories ÷ 4 or 9 = Grams
Example	*35%*	*1422 x 0.35 = 498*	*498 ÷ 4 = 125*
Carbohydrate	35%	x 0.35 =	÷ 4 =
Carbohydrate	40%	x 0.40 =	÷ 4 =
Protein	25%	x 0.25 =	÷ 4 =
Fat	35%	x 0.35 =	÷ 9 =
Fat	40%	x 0.40 =	÷ 9 =

Types of Exercises or Workouts that Fall Under Functional Movement & Flexibility:

1. Meditative or mindful yoga
2. Gardening or other household duties and chores
3. Bending, lifting, or carrying things on a daily basis, and going up and down steps
4. Group fitness classes—Pilates, yoga, yogalates, qigong, functional training (light intensity), foam rolling/stretching, barre (basic), and Tai Chi

MEAL BREAK-DOWN, TIMING & TRACKING:
For All Fitness Goals

Meal break-down: It is important to be consistent so you know what's working for you over a period of time. These calculations are super helpful for keeping you in check while meeting your fitness and nutritional goals, but *all* of these calculations are still estimations. Therefore, even when calculating and figuring out your BMR, some variances should be considered since these are all estimations.

Once you figure out how many calories you need in addition to your BMR, it is up to you to decide how you'd like to eat those calories throughout the day. I don't suggest eating all those calories in one or two large meals; instead, you should space out those calories throughout the day. I feel the best when I eat every two and a half to three hours, and I make sure that I don't go past four hours without eating. This plan works very well for me. Journaling and tracking how often you eat your meals are conducive to fine-tuning your best eating plan that works with your lifestyle.

I've learned to be very attuned to my body. I can feel when I need to eat and when my blood sugars are low. Pushing off my hunger when I think I'm too busy throws off my day, mood, and hormones. When you postpone eating or want to hold off because you think you're saving calories, the end result leads to overeating in the evening. By overeating, you're making up for calories not consumed during the day when your body can put them to good use. Listen to your own body and know what's best for it, even when tempted by things that lead you away from your goals. Set timers or reminders when to eat if you have to.

Your meal spacing can be as simple as dividing the number of meals you want to eat throughout the day by your total daily calorie goal. For example, if you need to eat 1600 calories and you want to eat five meals per day, each meal would be 320 calories. It's super simple, and there's no reason why you can't do it that way.

If you want to be more meticulous about the timing of your meals, the first thing you should do is focus on the timing of food around your workout, then go from there. Macronutrients all play a role in our nutritional success, and we can use them to maximize results!

Meal timing around exercise: I exercise first thing in the morning on a calorie-free liquid diet—black coffee, water, and a scoop of powder aminos to ensure my body has sufficient essential amino acids. I'm at the gym by 5 a.m. on most mornings and have become accustomed to the get up and go schedule. I have trained my body to perform and produce a great workout with exceptional results using this method.

You will find evidence that supports both eating and not eating before a morning workout. On the flip side, there are controversies to each case. It comes down to personal preference, performance, and the type of workout you're doing first thing in the morning. If you don't feel your best without eating, which negatively affects your workout in the morning, you should incorporate a meal before exercise. What happened with me is that I ended up eating less and less in the morning before I exercised until it came to the point that I just didn't have time to eat. I quickly adapted to not eating anything without my performance or energy output suffering. I found that the more conditioned I was, the better my body performed exercise without eating, which made it easier for me to implement my current method.

Depending on when you get up, you might not have enough time to sit down and make something, so drinking your calories may be a time-saving option. Low-fat smoothies or shakes would work best. Foods and shakes should be low in fiber, which is slow to digest; great for the middle of the day, but not right before a workout session.

Meal choice and size matter, depending on how much time there is between eating and exercising. If you eat two hours before you exercise, you can handle a mid-sized meal with a mix of complex and simple carbohydrates plus protein and low-to-moderate fat. If you eat less than an hour prior, then a grab-and-go meal of simple and low-fiber carbohydrates with a bit of protein and low fat is best. Fiber can cause an upset stomach because it is digested in the colon, and fat slows digestion—something else to avoid right before a workout.

Evening eating gets a bad rap because late eating tends to be in the form of junk food. Also, if you're one of those people who push off eating as long as you can during the day, you binge-eat at night. Let's kick that bad habit to the curb and assume you learned how to space your meals throughout the day, and you're now following one of my nutritional plans to reach your fitness goal.

If you were just at the gym lifting weights, out for a run, in a spin class, or any type of exercise, then why wouldn't you want to use food to replenish your body? It would be best to eat after a workout to promote protein synthesis, which is the process of creating protein molecules that contribute to making hormones, enzymes, new muscle, and replenishing glycogen stores.

If you're not adequately refueling your body with the essential macronutrients, you could potentially delay progress and compromise your following workout the next day. When it comes to your nutrition, not only are you planning for your body that day but the day after. What you do today affects you tomorrow. That's true for your food fuel, fitness activities, and life choices. Plan your day to maximize the effort you're putting into your training and eating. Then you can reap the benefits of your outcome.

Let's look at your nutrition plan as a whole. If you are eating within your set caloric parameters, the meal after your evening workout is already planned into your day. These are planned calories and should not cause you to gain weight. However, there are studies that state sleep and hormone disruption can occur when ingesting a bunch of carbohydrates. This disruption happened when a high amount of carbohydrates were included in the overall meal, and the subject went to sleep soon after.

That's why spacing out your meals and calories throughout the day is important. To avoid overeating at night, I suggest leaving about a two-hour buffer between your last big meal of the day and bedtime. Have some calories leftover after your last meal? Have a small snack before bed then, no problem!

Post-exercise meal timing—Does it matter? For your post-workout meal, research suggests that eating within a specific window of time after your workout is best for metabolism and absorption. That time varies from fifteen to sixty minutes. However, there is also supporting evidence that it doesn't matter if you eat within that prime time window, post-exercise, as long as you eat the right macronutrients by the end of the day.

I'll give you my take on it, and ultimately, you get to decide what works for you. This is, after all, *your* plan. That's what I'm freeing you from in the first place. When I eat my post-workout meal, I typically eat within forty-five to ninety minutes, but sometimes it's sooner, like twenty to thirty minutes. This variance is because I have small kids. After the gym, if I need to rush around getting them ready for the day, my needs typically take a backseat—just for a little while, though! So if I'm creeping up on that ninety-minute mark, mama needs to eat!

If I can help it, I want to take advantage of any anabolic window after I've damaged muscle tissue (in a good way!). This anabolic window typically occurs after strength training or TBC. If your workout lasts more than ninety minutes, then that window to replenish your muscle and glycogen stores should be shortly after your workout and should be a more extensive meal rather than a snack if your meal sizes differ. Getting proper nutrients into your body to initiate muscle rebuilding and restoring energy reserves sounds like a win to me!

Meal tracking: I've spent a lot of time discussing the importance of eating within a certain amount of calories and eating specific macronutrients within percentage ranges. Now it's time to talk about how exactly you're going to do that. Luckily, you don't have to use a pencil and paper to track your food in this day and age. Today, there are apps with large databases that can help you track.

Tracking what you eat is the only way to know if you're hitting your target percentages and calories. Guessing or half tracking usually fails to make the changes you need or want. So please don't go through the trouble of calculating your macros without tracking all of them. That's like going to the doctor for an illness, not taking the medication prescribed to cure it, and wondering why you're not better. You took the step to seek help but didn't follow through with all the steps to get better.

You can use any way to track that you want. For example, I use MyFitnessPal to track my macros, and many of my clients also use it. It's pretty user-friendly, even for the free version, which I also use. You can create a free account on your computer or download the app on your phone. You do not need to purchase the premium account to be able to change your calories and macros in your specific fitness goal range.

MyFitnessPal

[Scan QR Code] You can create a free account using www.myfitnesspal.com.

Tracking food and eating the measured amount of food will give you a great visual and a better understanding of what your daily calorie and macro targets look like and feel like to eat. If you are a visual person like myself, seeing the pie charts of my macronutrients puts what I'm eating in a better perspective. You will probably be surprised to see how many carbohydrates and fats are in certain foods. An eye-opening moment for many people is realizing the imbalance of their current eating habits before they start paying attention to their macro percentages.

Tracking your food isn't forever, but it is helpful whenever you need to tighten up or change your nutrition plan to reach another fitness goal. I know my foods pretty well—portion sizes and the macro breakdown of most foods—but I will still track my food when working towards a new fitness goal. I will usually track for a solid two weeks, and then I'm golden. The more you track, the easier it will be to make educated guesses about any foods you eat that you haven't prepared yourself.

Eating out can be challenging to track, especially proper portion sizes. So, if you have already been tracking and measuring out your food, it will be easier to recognize and estimate a cup of rice or pasta or roughly the number of ounces of protein on your plate.

Let me close with this about tracking: track everything you can! If you can't track something or don't have the exact ounces or amount, don't stress and obsess about it. After all, these numbers and formulas we are using to help our bodies are estimations, so why stress yourself out by needing to get the exact number on everything you track. What matters is that the food itself is recorded on your food log. Be sure to track your *bad* meals and any foods you'd consider junk. Learn to eat the macros you find the hardest to get early in the day, and make this a great learning experience to read food labels and gain knowledge about natural, whole foods.

My fitness transformation: I've used all of the methods I'm sharing with you to transform my body, taking it as far as competing in bodybuilding, fitness, and figure. Now that's a transformation like nothing before! First, I kept my calories a little over my BMR when I trained. Then, I focused on my macro percentages and exercises and relied on that to drop body fat to where I needed it to step on stage. The key takeaway is that I *did not* starve myself to get where I needed to be!

When I started my training journey to compete, I had already been working out pretty regularly for about a year because I was unhappy with where my less active, crazy eating patterns had led me during my sophomore year in college. So my husband (boyfriend at the time) and I decided to join a weight loss challenge to feel more like ourselves again.

Growing up, I was very active and never had any issues with my weight. However, I really noticed the change in my shape and weight going into my second year of college. My body composition was my biggest concern. My body fat had crept up to somewhere in the upper twenties or low thirties, and I was losing the muscle tone I had developed through sports.

When I decided to compete, I had worked hard all year to drop fifteen pounds and reduce my body fat to the low twenties. Focused and driven, I was able to drop my body fat down to around ten percent to compete in my first figure competition in 2007.

During my transformation journey, I found my passion and love for fitness and nutrition. So, making the connection between food-fueled workouts and what our magnificent bodies are capable of doing, I switched my major at Penn State University to Kinesiology/Exercise Science—and the rest was history!

METHOD # 5:
Water, Hydration Needs, & Water Jug Challenge

Water is such a big piece of the puzzle, but we often overlook it and don't place a high value on it. You're thinking, "I really need to drink more water," but you never put that thought into action. It will remain a thought until the day you actually start charting and start doing something different from your normal day-to-day activities—why? Because water isn't and hasn't been a part of your daily routine for so long, you're not bothered by not drinking enough water to make that change. Instead, you need to be intentional about it and take action.

A general guideline for water was put out there for people to refer to—*The 8x8 Rule*—drink eight 8-ounce glasses of water a day. The 8x8 rule will get you to sixty-four ounces of water per day. If you weigh about 128 pounds, that should get you to your recommended water intake. But, for me, sixty-four ounces is not enough; then, add some vigorous exercise that makes me sweat, and I'm even further away from my water intake goal.

How much a physically active person should drink varies greatly. Some sports medicine organizations have created their own guidelines for athletes based on contemporary research. Still, these organizations' recommendations vary from one another. In rare cases, you may hear

about athletes overhydrating, which can end in disaster. So what guidelines should you use, and what should you be drinking?

If you hardly drink any water, a good start would be incorporating two to three cups of water a day. For some people, you have already consumed that much water by mid-morning, and for others, it will be a stretch to get it in before bedtime. If you're not a water drinker, the goal is to form this new habit so that consuming water will not feel forced.

For hydration simplicity, you can use the *urine test* as a hydration guide. The lighter in color your urine is, the more hydrated you are. Not to be gross, but did you ever take a look in the toilet in the morning after a night of drinking some alcoholic beverages? If you didn't drink much water between beverages, that toilet bowl has some golden liquid inside. Dehydration is a significant contributor to hangover headaches the next day!

When using the urine test method, keep track of how many ounces of water/liquid you're drinking during the day. It is normal to wake up in the yellow-to-dark yellow urine range, but the idea is to drink enough liquids to move to the light yellow-to-clear urine range during the day leading into the evening. Then, figure out a good water intake cut-off time so you're not disrupting your precious sleep by bathroom breaks during the night.

I use another hydration method that works very well for me and many of my clients—*the divide by two method*. For active individuals, take your current body weight, divide it by two, and that's how many ounces of water you should consume daily. For example, if you weigh 160 pounds, your water intake is 80 ounces. Of course, your water intake should change when your body weight changes. If you add environmental factors like heat and humidity that increase your sweat rate, you could drink closer to an ounce for every pound you weigh.

By now, I hope you've noticed one of the most significant differences between my recommendations and other traditional diets. What makes my nutritional plans successful is that *your* body weight and the calculated numbers specific to *you* matter. How much to eat and drink should be based on your current status and not just some number someone told you to shoot for. If you know someone trying out a diet that gives generic numbers that have nothing to do with their body or fitness goal, I challenge you to ask them—why? Where are the numbers coming from, and will those numbers and type of diet work with their body to maximize results?

If you tend to do very strenuous exercises and you feel that you sweat a lot, water alone might not cut it, especially if you experience any muscle cramping. When you sweat, you lose sodium, and by adding water, you can further dilute the sodium-potassium balance. Drinking electrolytes or coconut water can help rehydrate and restore balance. Hydrating beverages or electrolyte powders or drinks count towards your total water intake. I look for lower sugar drinks and stick to things for the intended purpose—to hydrate and restore. High sugar recovery drinks are rarely necessary for the average person; they add unnecessary calories that you are working so hard to burn off anyway.

I get asked a lot about what counts towards water or liquid consumption. Depending on who you talk to, you will get various answers, just like the differences of opinion on water intake. I include seltzer and carbonated water, flavored or infused water, juice, milk, almond milk, oat milk, coconut milk, homemade hot or cold tea, and broth in my total water consumption for the day. You could argue coffee and highly caffeinated tea are water-based and could count towards your daily intake—I don't. My answer is as simple as that. Nor do I count sodas, hard seltzers, slushies, or other sugary drinks you'd find at the store.

We live in a fast-paced world, and we are busy all the time. I frequently hear from clients that they are so busy during the day or at their job that they forget to drink. This new habit of increasing your water and liquid intake can be pretty hard to form if you're too busy to slow down and drink. Out of sight, out of mind is a real thing! In my experience, when clients have told me they think they will start drinking more water, the reality is they continually fail to put that thought into action. So I enforced the water jug challenge as their visual and action step.

What is the water jug challenge? The water jug (not chug!) challenge is our best hydration accountability partner. If you're using the divide by two method, you already have the number of ounces to shoot for. This challenge is so effective because it gives you a visual of your total water intake, and who doesn't love a little friendly competition against a jug or container? There is no way you're letting that water jug win! Materials needed for this challenge are:

- o Gallon water jug, pitcher, or container able to hold your daily water intake

- o   Permanent markers, paint, stickers, etcetera
- o   A little creativity (but not much)

Mark a *fill line* on the container of your choice so you know how much to fill it each day. To find where you should mark the fill line, showing the number of ounces, take your current weight and divide it by two. Unfortunately, gallon jugs don't provide hash marks, so the easiest way is to start with an empty jug and fill it up to the pre-determined ounce level using a liquid measuring cup. Be sure to use a liquid measuring cup and not a measuring cup for dry ingredients! (Side note: My mom and stepdad are bakers, and that type of rookie mistake could get you in a lot of trouble!)

The rest of the lines and creativity on the jug are pretty much up to you. You can evenly space hash marks down the jug to the bottom and write little sayings at each hash mark like, "keep chuggin'" or "you got this." Feel free to doodle or write motivating or funny phrases on your jug to make the jug *yours*.

Carry the jug with you everywhere you go. If you leave it behind, you're missing out on the opportunity to kick some H2O butt! Of course, if you'd prefer to pour the water out of your jug into something smaller to drink from, that is perfectly fine. You can also use the water from your container to make your tea, protein shake, or mix up your powdered supplements.

Have your jug visible at all times. Set the jug or pitcher out on your counter, desk, or wherever you are so you can see the water as a reminder. There is nothing else that will make your water disappear except for you. (P.S. don't let anyone else drink from your jug. Also, pace yourself throughout the day, so you're not left with more than half of your water to finish at dinner time.)

The water jug challenge genuinely does help, and soon you will be feeling hydrated and energetic! Also, if you've been hitting the gym regularly and haven't been getting the right amount of water you need, you will likely feel the difference in your performance and recovery. So, yes, water is that important and makes a big difference!

The fitness challenges I created were about more than just weight loss. They focused on overall lifestyle changes and body composition. For example, I decided to start the first week of my fitness challenge with the water jug challenge. Though I didn't invent this challenge, I adapted the idea and set up guidelines that fit my own teachable fitness principles.

There was a twenty-something-year-old female who joined my fitness challenge in hopes of losing inches and bloat. She wasn't overweight but was a little thicker in the middle. Her body composition could be improved by reducing her body fat slightly, but honestly, she was in decent shape.

Usually, when people hear the word bloat, they immediately think, "I should eliminate carbohydrates or dairy." However, based on her dietary habits and daily food choices, I wasn't convinced it all had to do with her diet and exercise. Together, we set her target water/liquid intake for the day and made it official on her jug.

Even though her water consumption wasn't the only new adjustment to her plan, that is what she had focused on the most. She ate relatively the same types of foods as she did before the challenge, except for increasing her protein intake. She was the type of person who couldn't handle many changes at once, and that was perfectly fine.

On this journey, it's okay to start with one habit change at a time. Some people like to make dramatic changes at once—*all or nothing* personalities. Others crumble before they even begin because the idea of many new changes all at once is too overwhelming. I suggest starting with one to two new changes in your lifestyle at a time; this is where I see that people have the most success.

Within two weeks, my female client had seen a dramatic change in the way she looked and felt, even though the scale didn't show any drastic changes. She lost about a pound and a half, which is definitely a win in a two-week span. Yet, her biggest and best achievement was that her bloat was completely gone!

As we continued through the last four weeks of the challenge, she stayed dedicated to her water and fluid intake as well as her exercise. At times, she struggled to meet her protein needs throughout the week, but overall, she stayed very close to the macros that fit best with her fitness goal.

She was absolutely amazed about changing something that seemed so insignificant, like water, and how that small change positively affected so many things in her body. She reported having clearer, nicer skin, a more controlled appetite, was more energetic, eliminated bloat, and lost almost five inches on her waist and hips during the challenge.

She was a perfect example of starting with one small lifestyle change that saved time and aggravation regarding a problem that stemmed from something as simple as keeping track of her daily water and liquid consumption.

Before you jump to conclusions about your personal theories of why you're feeling a certain way or don't feel like you're operating at 100 percent, it's not a bad idea to start with some of the basics before you do something more drastic, like cutting certain foods out of your diet because you think they are negatively affecting you.

Divide by Two Hydration Method

*Multiple equations are provided if weight changes every four to six weeks

Date:_____ Current weight:_____(lbs) ÷ 2 = _____(oz water)

Date:_____ Current weight:_____(lbs) ÷ 2 = _____(oz water)

Date:_____ Current weight:_____(lbs) ÷ 2 = _____(oz water)

Date:_____ Current weight:_____(lbs) ÷ 2 = _____(oz water)

METHOD # 6:
Bring Your Fitness & Nutrition Goals Home—and Everywhere Else for that Matter!

It's time to bring your fitness and nutrition goals home and live them out in your day-to-day routine. I don't mean quit the gym, if you belong to one, and start working out at home. I mean, your fitness goals and efforts should not be left at the gym in some stinky locker, like a pair of shoes you will put on the next day to work out. Connecting your fitness life, family life, work life, and social life will help bring your fitness and nutrition goals to fruition and help you achieve what you want.

If you abandon the goals you are striving towards in social gatherings, at home or work life, or with people closest to you, you will never make the changes necessary to create new habits. It's almost like you are wrestling with two identities—one who you wish you were and one who you are right now. You will only get to live out both identities if you start intertwining the two.

Remember that my book aims to empower others—to make eating and exercise as enjoyable as possible while being the best version of yourself and putting this power back in your control. *YOU* are the reason I wrote this book. You also have an essential role in my story—influencing and inspiring people you interact with, starting with the people closest to you in your home and then branching out from there.

Don't underestimate the power of your influence on others. We are influential people, and living life together is what we were meant to do. We weren't built to have it all, but sharing stories, tips, struggles, and victories with the people around us makes us stronger together.

A while back, I read a book about successful leadership skills, and there was something written that resonated with me. It stated that in order to be successful, you must focus on your strengths not your weaknesses to become a strong leader. What was written wasn't about leveling up your weaknesses but was about developing your strengths and leaning into what you are naturally good at instead of wasting time on something you were never meant to be. In addition, sharing your goals and living out your desires to change with people you interact with daily can help you succeed.

Your weakness is another's strength. Maybe your weakness is social temptation. That strong-willed friend of yours will help you stay the course in a social gathering and karate-kick anything that gets in your way. Or maybe you cannot survive without an accountability partner at home and in the gym. Or you can't cook, but you found out that a co-worker is a fantastic, healthy cook who will now share simple recipes you can follow and make for your family every week.

People naturally shine when asked to do something they are good at or feel very passionate about. Let your circle of people lend you their strengths if that's an area of weakness for you, especially if it wastes too much time and energy. Don't forget that you have your own strengths to share with others, so pay it forward when you are called to shine.

PLATEAUS ARE ACTUALLY GOOD

Let's be honest; it can be pretty easy to lose your drive, even your purpose, if you're not intentionally thinking or working towards anything. I see this all of the time with people. So I'm going to bring out the big "P" word—*plateau.* The word plateau gets a bad rap, and people think they've hit one even when they didn't because we, as a society, are impatient and want change to happen quickly.

A plateau is your body telling you that it's ready for another change. A true plateau is when your body has made zero change or progress for about four weeks. So don't freak out if a week or two goes by without change; that doesn't mean you've plateaued and need to change everything you're doing.

When I see people at the gym doing the same exercise routine, using the same weight week after week with no changes, the routine will eventually run its course. Our bodies were made to adapt, and they are doing just that! I like using the word *stale* in describing these types of plateaus in the fitness and nutrition world.

Have you ever made bread? It can be a lengthy process, depending on the bread type, the yeast and flour mixtures, and the rising time. The initial work you put into your eating plan and workouts can take a while as you get acquainted with tracking your macros or understanding the exercises and form. This process can be different for each individual. Clients I previously worked with had all different learning abilities and skill levels. The time needed until they mastered their eating plan or felt confident in their choices ranged from a week to a month. That is okay!

Back to my analogy between stale routines and stale bread: After you have put in the work to make the bread, it's ready to go in the oven and bake. That smell of freshly made bread excites all of my senses. Cutting into that bread with the chewy, crunchy crust and doughy center is unbelievable! That's similar to the point in your program where you start reaping the benefits of your new nutrition and fitness plan.

Okay, let's recap. You figured out your fitness goal and nutrition plan. It's a process; some people need more time than others for this process, and the same is true for making bread. There is no right or wrong time frame you need to follow, as long as you get there! You are seeing changes; things are going well. But then, suddenly, you haven't made any progress for four weeks. From the bread you made, there's a two-inch-thick piece left from the end that's been sitting on your counter in a zip-lock.

You can do one of two things if you want more bread (or more results). You can chuck it and start with a new recipe. (Remember, it can sometimes be a process to make.) Or you can reuse or tweak the bread—chop it up, and put it in the oven to make croutons. Either way, we need to do something different with the stale bread on the counter, or it will get moldy and disgusting. Please! I would never call you moldy or disgusting, but you get my point. Plateaus happen, so let's be ready for them!

LIVING YOUR BEST LIFE

I'm going to close with this: It is worth every second to put time and effort into your nutrition and fitness. You are worth the energy spent putting the right foods in your body, moving with ease, being healthy enough to avoid medications, and living life to its fullest.

This is a fast-paced world we live in. I'm guilty of being on the go a lot, but not to the point where I need to sacrifice my health or fitness goals. We are a sleepless society, and we can only go for so long until we break down. Sleep and your overall well-being will influence your results. Remember when I talked about BMR and told you if you're not giving your body enough calories, it will struggle to change because its needs are not being met? Sleep is a need.

Please don't claim that you don't need sleep because you do. You have just learned to function (or half function) on lack of sleep. Getting less than seven to nine hours of sleep a night can have consequences that hinder your progress. Even though hours of sleep are something we can usually control, people let this one slip from their top priorities. Recall that you are working on living out your best life, so let's get to it!

Not getting enough shut-eye can cause unclear thinking or trouble concentrating, weaken your immune system, increase your risk for disease, and mess up cell signaling. All of these can lead to weight gain and negatively affect hormone balance. However, you have the power to make changes in your schedule for better nutrition, fitness, and sleep.

You may play catch-up on sleep within a few days of coming up shy of what you need by sleeping longer a night or two after missed sleep. Power naps can work, too, to help recharge the body. I caution you, however, not to rely on power naps throughout your week if you are cutting into your sleep-time night after night while you're up late playing video games, on your phone, or watching television. Naps and more extended periods of sleep can be helpful when they are needed but shouldn't be depended upon. And no, the sleep you missed last week cannot be made up a week or more afterward—it's just gone!

Ever since I have intentionally prioritized my nutrition and fitness, it has positively influenced how I feel and live every day. Being intuitive about my daily fitness and nutrition is second nature. I love being a positive influence on my family, and we have all joined forces to live our lives to the fullest. Living our best life comes down to our daily choices, the people we surround ourselves with, and the happiness we get to share with one another. But, like anything else, it takes work.

I'm so excited for you to take this into your own hands! *Act As If.* .you completely understand everything I laid out for you in this book. Keep acting until you start doing, and keep doing until you believe it can be achieved. Then you *will* achieve it!

APPENDIX A:
Dani's Food Go-To's

Here's a little insight on putting together meals and snacks: Combining carbohydrates and proteins often causes you to feel full and satisfied because carbs provide your body with energy, and protein increases satiety. Eating a combination of protein plus carbs after resistance training or endurance workouts helps stimulate muscle repair and growth. In addition, fat and fiber make your stomach empty more slowly, which helps reduce the glycemic response (blood sugar and insulin spike) after a meal.

I put together a list of foods that are my favorite go-to's. You'll see that the list is separated by macronutrient, and I've added notes to help you. It's great to use as a reference when you go grocery shopping. Also, just because certain foods you eat are not on my list doesn't mean it's off-limits (because nothing really is), but this is me sharing what I eat with you! Use my list to get started with your own. I have provided space for you to create your own list of *go-to's* in Appendix B. Categorize the healthy foods you like to eat by macronutrients. Your list can be very similar to mine. Make substitutions for foods I have on my list that better fit your eating style. For example, if you're a vegetarian or don't eat dairy products. The foods that end up on your list should be nutritious, and for the most part, minimally processed. When you base most of your meals from foods off your list, you can feel good knowing that most of your daily meals are healthy and nutritious when you do indulge in some of your favorite *not so healthy* foods!

CARBOHYDRATES	DANI'S NOTES
Oatmeal & oatmeal cups	I usually buy quick oats. RX brand oatmeal cups are perfect meals for on the go
Beans (black, garbanzo, kidney)	Always have them on-hand
Wasa crackers	One-ingredient crackers! Great to top with tuna or chicken for lunch
Quinoa	I make large batches ahead of time to make many meals. I eat it cold or hot
Rice cakes	I eat all flavors—sweet and savory, small and large. I love topping them or dipping them
Brown, basmati, or jasmine rice	I make large batches and use leftovers to make a bunch of different ways
Fruit preserves	I mix it in with my Greek yogurt, cottage cheese, or use as a topper for a rice cake PB & J

CARBOHYDRATES	DANI'S NOTES
Potatoes: white, gold, red, sweet potatoes, yams	I bake them in the oven for dinner and dice in the morning for breakfast. I also love eating sweet potatoes cold the next day, don't knock it until you've tried it!
Protein pasta or whole-grain pasta	Have it on hand, and eat it a couple of times a month
Black bean, chickpea, edamame pasta	This pasta is packed with protein. I use this for meatless meals
Vegetables - Broccoli, asparagus, string beans, cauliflower, peppers, onions, mushrooms, Brussel sprouts, zucchini, cucumbers, cabbage, carrots, celery, beets	These are my favorite veggies to snack on and mix in with meals, and always have on hand
Canned pumpkin (not pumpkin pie)	I make pumpkin pancakes, oatmeal, and homemade lattes all year round; pumpkin is not just for fall
Salad greens: Lettuce, spinach, kale, arugula	I like to use them in salads or cooked with meals

CARBOHYDRATES	DANI'S NOTES
Fruit: Apple, berries, grapefruit, orange, peach, pear, banana, grapes, kiwi, mango, lemon, lime, pineapple	I'll add fruit to meals. It's a healthy carb option to eat with protein or fat
Honey	Use in my tea when I'm sick or to lightly sweeten dishes when cooking/baking
Dates	I eat them with peanut butter. It's a small, but mighty snack
Cow milk, almond milk, and coconut milk	I use all kinds of milk when cooking, on my cereal, or in shakes.
Whole grain/protein cereals	One of my favorite mid-day or evening snacks
Protein waffles (store-bought or pre-made and stored in the freezer)	I like to have these on hand for a quick on-the-go option. Save calories and skip the butter and syrup; I top it with whipped cream
Whole wheat or Sourdough bread	I eat bread sparingly. Definitely watch portions
Soups: all varieties, low sodium	I love making bone broth-based soups, especially in fall/winter

PROTEINS	DANI'S NOTES
Chicken: Breast, ground, thighs, wings, canned	Use recipes to transform your boring chicken meals
Turkey: Breast, tenderloin, thighs, ground	I always have it on hand in the fridge or freezer to make meals. It's very versatile
Lean steak	When choosing a steak, look for less marbling, leaner cuts to eat
Pork	My favorite way to make all cuts of pork is in the crockpot
Fish: Mahi-mahi, tuna, salmon, shrimp, scallops	There's much more out there, but when it comes to seafood, I generally stick with these options
Eggs	Hard-boiled eggs are great for snacking. I eat eggs any time of the day. I love mixing egg whites in my oatmeal for a little protein boost
Edamame	I eat them cold or warm. Great to add to dishes and salads
Cottage cheese	Great mid-day snack with fruit preserves or fruit

PROTEINS	DANI'S NOTES
Greek yogurt	It's high in protein and has less sugar than regular yogurt. Regular and Greek yogurt both provide calcium and probiotics. I eat it as is or mix it into dishes to make them creamy, or I dip my rice cakes into it
Low-fat cheese and hard cheese	Portion control is the biggest concern with cheese. Check serving sizes when snacking
Bone Broth	I switched to bone broth instead of stock for added protein and lower sodium options. It's also great for sipping

FATS	DANI'S NOTES
Olive, Avocado, or Flaxseed oil	Use them for cooking or drizzling on roasted vegetables
Coconut oil	I often substitute this when recipes call for oil or butter. I also use it for makeup remover, and body moisturizer
Avocado	I add it to many dishes or use it to make a base for chocolate pudding

FATS	DANI'S NOTES
Peanut Butter, almond butter	Put it on rice cakes, carrots, or celery, or just eat it as is
PB2 (powdered peanut butter)	It's a low-fat peanut butter option to mix in shakes, Greek yogurt, or water
Nuts and seeds	I measure a serving to add to meals or snacks to compliment a carb, protein, or both!

MEAL ADD-ONS	DANI'S NOTES
Hummus	Great for dipping, topping, or spreads
Vinegars: balsamic, apple cider, white	Cook with it and use on salads
Ketchup	I opt for a lower sugar option if I use it; I'd rather use mustard
Mustards (all varieties)	All the mustard! I put it on most meats and tuna
Hot Sauce (low sodium)	I love a little spice with my meals
Liquid Aminos (tastes like soy sauce) or low sodium soy sauce	I use to make homemade Chinese or Asian inspired meals

MEAL ADD-ONS	DANI'S NOTES
Tomato Sauce (low sugar/sodium)	Watch out for sugar and sodium-loaded sauces. I always keep on hand
Salsa	It's always in my fridge
Yogurt-based dressings	Great for dipping and making healthier dips
Alcohol	I track it like I would anything else. I do not count alcohol towards my fluid intake. I track alcohol calories, but I don't replace any of the carbs from alcohol with the carbs needed in my macro plan
Coffee and tea	I drink these daily, as is; no cream or sugar. There are benefits to caffeine, but it has an upper limit of around 400 mg daily.

APPENDIX B:
My Food Go-To's

CARBOHYDRATES	MY NOTES

My Food Go-To's

PROTEINS	MY NOTES

FATS	MY NOTES

My Food Go-To's

MEAL ADD-ON	MY NOTES

My Food Go-To's
